# MY FITNESS TRACKER

## A JOURNAL TO HELP YOU MAP OUT AND IMPROVE YOUR HEALTH AND WELL-BEING

ANNA BARNES

MY FITNESS TRACKER

Copyright © Summersdale Publishers Ltd, 2022

All rights reserved.

Text by Kitiara Pascoe

No part of this book may be reproduced by any means, nor transmitted, nor translated into a machine language, without the written permission of the publishers.

Condition of Sale
This book is sold subject to the condition that it shall not, by way of trade or otherwise, be lent, resold, hired out or otherwise circulated in any form of binding or cover other than that in which it is published and without a similar condition including this condition being imposed on the subsequent purchaser.

An Hachette UK Company
www.hachette.co.uk

Vie Books, an imprint of Summersdale Publishers Ltd
Part of Octopus Publishing Group Limited
Carmelite House
50 Victoria Embankment
LONDON
EC4Y 0DZ
UK

www.summersdale.com

Printed and bound in China

ISBN: 978-1-80007-448-4

Substantial discounts on bulk quantities of Summersdale books are available to corporations, professional associations and other organizations. For details contact general enquiries: telephone: +44 (0) 1243 771107 or email: enquiries@summersdale.com.

## Disclaimer

This book is not intended as a substitute for the medical advice of a doctor or physician. If you are experiencing problems with your health, it is always best to follow the advice of a medical professional.

# Introduction

Do you want to kick your health and well-being into gear but can't decide where to start? What should you focus on? Where will the time come from? The last thing you want is to feel stressed about improving your health. Don't worry, you've come to the right place.

When we keep our bodies fit and healthy, we give ourselves the best possible chance at getting the most from life and facing any challenges that come our way. While it's easy to view parts of the body in isolation, there's no doubt that everything within us is connected.

For instance, eating healthily fuels our muscles and brains, allowing us to move smoothly and think clearly, and being active sends oxygen more efficiently through our bodies, making exercise easier and improving our overall health. The food we consume affects our hormones and our energy levels – when we fill our plates with colourful vegetables, healthy fats and fibre-filled wholegrain, we're giving our bodies exactly what they need to thrive.

And what of the mind? Staying fit and eating well aids our sleep, which gives us an ideal base from which to start our day. Challenging ourselves with fitness pursuits also builds confidence and self-esteem.

Our minds and bodies are complex and ever-changing, as are our priorities. When you track your health and fitness, you can see patterns, set yourself new goals and reflect on your progress. This journal is here to support your physical and mental health, allowing you to track your exercise, weight, intake of fruit and vegetables, water and alcohol, and general wellness. Each month, you can set goals and map out your progress, flick through the tips whenever you need a bit of inspiration and try out the affirmations when you need some motivation.

Turn the page to begin your journey…

# Exercise Tracker

Using the key, colour in and add patterns to the trainers in the space below to help you gauge how much exercise you're doing. If you feel like you're smashing it, then keep up the good work. But if you think you could do better, there's always next month!

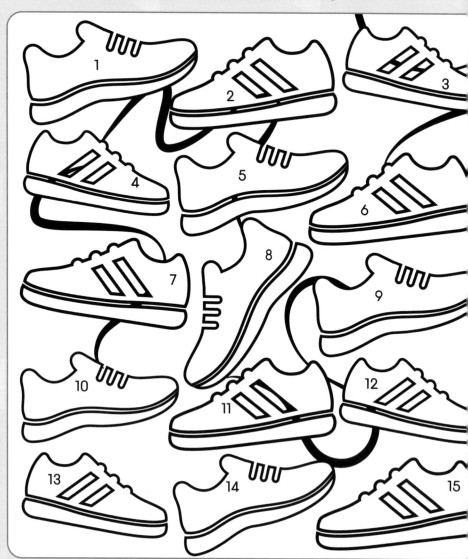

# KEY

 less than 30 mins

 30–60 mins

 60+ mins

 cardio

 stretching

strengthening/ toning

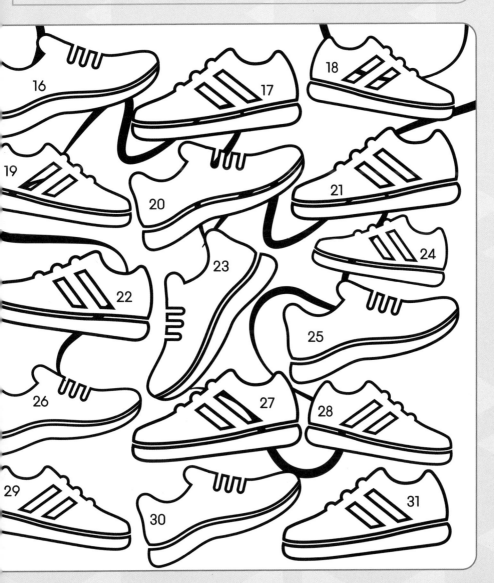

I AM WHAT
I CHOOSE
TO BE

# TOP TIPS

## FIND A FRIEND

It's easy to talk ourselves out of getting some exercise, but letting a friend down? That's much harder. Whether you're building your fitness in a particular sport or you want to try new exercise classes or activities, a great way to stay motivated is to get a friend on board to keep you on track.

The two (or more) of you can make plans to meet every week for classes, runs, bike rides or gym sessions – whatever you fancy. If you don't live near each other, no sweat. You can still set fitness goals together and send each other motivating messages. And, of course, a sweaty selfie (no filter required) is fun proof that you are achieving your goals.

Sharing your fitness journey with a friend guarantees laughs and builds your friendship – and, as well as reaching your own fitness goals, you get the extra bonus of knowing you're helping someone you love reach their goals too.

# Five-a-Day Tracker

Each apple = one of your five fruits or vegetables a day

1 🍎🍎🍎🍎🍎🍎
2 🍎🍎🍎🍎🍎🍎
3 🍎🍎🍎🍎🍎🍎
4 🍎🍎🍎🍎🍎🍎
5 🍎🍎🍎🍎🍎🍎
6 🍎🍎🍎🍎🍎🍎
7 🍎🍎🍎🍎🍎🍎
8 🍎🍎🍎🍎🍎🍎
9 🍎🍎🍎🍎🍎🍎
10 🍎🍎🍎🍎🍎🍎
11 🍎🍎🍎🍎🍎🍎
12 🍎🍎🍎🍎🍎🍎
13 🍎🍎🍎🍎🍎🍎
14 🍎🍎🍎🍎🍎🍎
15 🍎🍎🍎🍎🍎🍎

16 🍎🍎🍎🍎🍎🍎
17 🍎🍎🍎🍎🍎🍎
18 🍎🍎🍎🍎🍎🍎
19 🍎🍎🍎🍎🍎🍎
20 🍎🍎🍎🍎🍎🍎
21 🍎🍎🍎🍎🍎🍎
22 🍎🍎🍎🍎🍎🍎
23 🍎🍎🍎🍎🍎🍎
24 🍎🍎🍎🍎🍎🍎
25 🍎🍎🍎🍎🍎🍎
26 🍎🍎🍎🍎🍎🍎
27 🍎🍎🍎🍎🍎🍎
28 🍎🍎🍎🍎🍎🍎
29 🍎🍎🍎🍎🍎🍎
30 🍎🍎🍎🍎🍎🍎
31 🍎🍎🍎🍎🍎🍎

# My Goals and Achievements

Don't worry if you don't manage to achieve your goals —
any progress is great and there's always next month!

## My goal(s) for this month

Example goal: Do a yoga class twice a week

- ........................................................  **ACHIEVED Y/N**

- ........................................................  **ACHIEVED Y/N**

- ........................................................  **ACHIEVED Y/N**

## Steps to make the goal(s) achievable

Example steps: Pick a studio and/or online class that suits
my fitness level and schedule; set a reminder in phone/
diary; have my yoga gear ready the evening before

- ........................................................

........................................................

- ........................................................

........................................................

- ........................................................

........................................................

# Healthy Weight Tracker

Keeping track of your weight doesn't need to fill you with dread as long as you remind yourself that the figures that appear on the scales are just one part of your healthy body maintenance. Weight fluctuations occur throughout the day and can be caused by many factors including hormone levels, so don't worry about small increases or decreases. The most important information you want to keep track of is your BMI, as this shows you whether you are a healthy weight for your height.

Try to weigh yourself on the same day at the same time each week.

Don't scrutinize the small numbers; maintaining a healthy lifestyle is what's most important.

|        | Week One | Week Two | Week Three | Week Four |
|--------|----------|----------|------------|-----------|
| Weight |          |          |            |           |
| BMI    |          |          |            |           |
| Chest  |          |          |            |           |
| Waist  |          |          |            |           |
| Hips   |          |          |            |           |

To work out your BMI, calculate your weight divided by your height squared (in metric). Find the BMI chart on page 152 to see the results of your BMI.

# Water Tracker

One drop = one glass (400 ml)

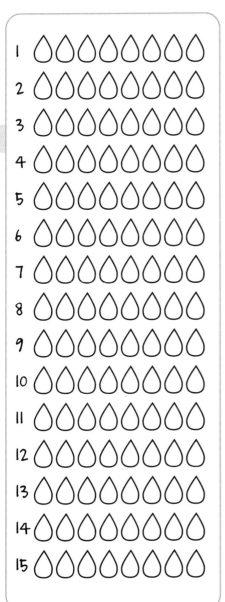

1  ○○○○○○○○
2  ○○○○○○○○
3  ○○○○○○○○
4  ○○○○○○○○
5  ○○○○○○○○
6  ○○○○○○○○
7  ○○○○○○○○
8  ○○○○○○○○
9  ○○○○○○○○
10 ○○○○○○○○
11 ○○○○○○○○
12 ○○○○○○○○
13 ○○○○○○○○
14 ○○○○○○○○
15 ○○○○○○○○

16 ○○○○○○○○
17 ○○○○○○○○
18 ○○○○○○○○
19 ○○○○○○○○
20 ○○○○○○○○
21 ○○○○○○○○
22 ○○○○○○○○
23 ○○○○○○○○
24 ○○○○○○○○
25 ○○○○○○○○
26 ○○○○○○○○
27 ○○○○○○○○
28 ○○○○○○○○
29 ○○○○○○○○
30 ○○○○○○○○
31 ○○○○○○○○

# Alcohol Tracker

## One glass = one unit (recommended weekly intake: no more than 14 units)

Single shot of spirits (25 ml) = 1 unit
Alcopop (275 ml) = 1.5 units
Small glass of wine (125 ml) = 1.5 units
Pint of lower-strength lager/beer/cider
(ABV 3.6%) = 2 units

Standard glass of wine (175 ml) = 2.1 units
Pint of higher-strength lager/beer/cider
(ABV 5.2%) = 3 units
Large glass of wine (250 ml) = 3 units

# Wellness Tracker

On each day this month, colour in one
shape according to how you feel.

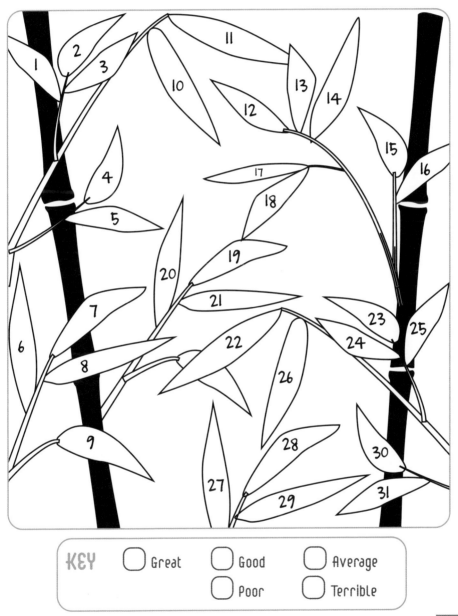

KEY
- ◯ Great
- ◯ Good
- ◯ Average
- ◯ Poor
- ◯ Terrible

Instead of believing in your limitations, start believing in yourself.

JAY SHETTY

# TOP TIPS

## FIND YOUR WHY

We've all been there. We feel a burst of motivation, make big decisions and set bold goals. This is great! That is, until we find ourselves a week later struggling to find that same drive. When the going gets tough, and it often does, we need to remind ourselves of the reasons we set these goals in the first place – why we booked a 7 a.m. spin class when bed is oh-so-comfy.

When you set a goal or start a new activity, take a moment to write down the reasons why you want to do it. Be as specific as possible. If you write, "I want to get fit," then it's easy to hit the snooze button because it lacks a specific "why". Instead, a stronger reason might be, "I want to do a spin workout twice a week so I can take my daughter cycling in the forest and not get too tired."

# Exercise Tracker

Using the key, colour in and add patterns to the trainers in the space below to help you gauge how much exercise you're doing. If you feel like you're smashing it, then keep up the good work. But if you think you could do better, there's always next month!

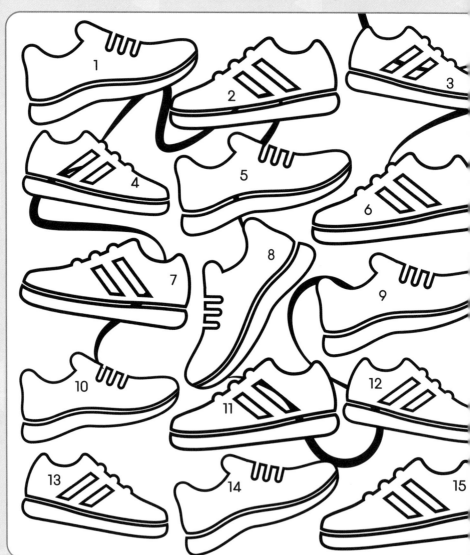

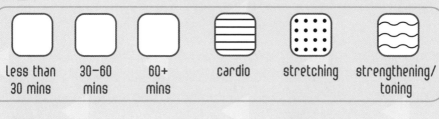

less than 30 mins | 30–60 mins | 60+ mins | cardio | stretching | strengthening/toning

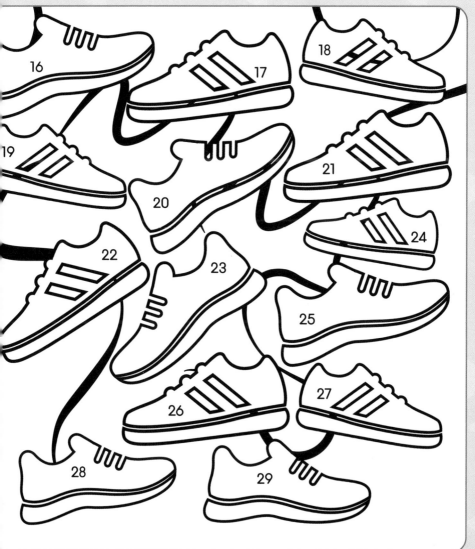

# MY POTENTIAL IS LIMITLESS

# TOP TIPS

## POWER YOURSELF

One of the easiest ways to become more active doesn't require a gym card or a weekly club: simply choose to be human-powered at every opportunity. This means walking, scootering or cycling whenever you get the chance. Here are some ideas:

- Walk or cycle to work.

- Take the stairs.

- Get a rucksack or bicycle panniers and head to the supermarket without your car.

- Take walking meetings outdoors whether in person or on the phone.

- During your lunch break, walk to a café or a park or just take a gentle stroll.

- Cycle or scoot for your errands, to your child's school or to see a friend.

Powering yourself on these kinds of journeys is a wonderful way to get exercise without even thinking about it. Plus, you're saving on fuel, preventing needless wear and tear on your car and reducing your environmental impact.

# Five-a-Day Tracker

Each apple = one of your five fruits or vegetables a day

# My Goals and Achievements

Don't worry if you don't manage to achieve your goals —
any progress is great and there's always next month!

## My goal(s) for this month

Example goal: Take part in a parkrun event

- ................................................................. **ACHIEVED Y/N**
- ................................................................. **ACHIEVED Y/N**
- ................................................................. **ACHIEVED Y/N**

## Steps to make the goal(s) achievable

Example steps: Find a local parkrun event; register
on parkrun.org.uk; prepare my running kit and
parkrun barcode the evening before

- .................................................................
  .................................................................
- .................................................................
  .................................................................
- .................................................................
  .................................................................

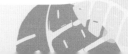

23

# Healthy Weight Tracker

Keeping track of your weight doesn't need to fill you with dread as long as you remind yourself that the figures that appear on the scales are just one part of your healthy body maintenance. Weight fluctuations occur throughout the day and can be caused by many factors including hormone levels, so don't worry about small increases or decreases. The most important information you want to keep track of is your BMI, as this shows you whether you are a healthy weight for your height.

> Try to weigh yourself on the same day at the same time each week.

> Don't scrutinize the small numbers; maintaining a healthy lifestyle is what's most important.

|        | Week One | Week Two | Week Three | Week Four |
|--------|----------|----------|------------|-----------|
| Weight |          |          |            |           |
| BMI    |          |          |            |           |
| Chest  |          |          |            |           |
| Waist  |          |          |            |           |
| Hips   |          |          |            |           |

To work out your BMI, calculate your weight divided by your height squared (in metric). Find the BMI chart on page 152 to see the results of your BMI.

# Water Tracker

One drop = one glass (400 ml)

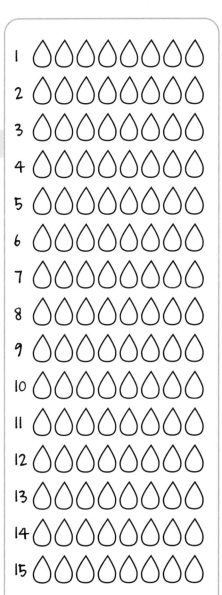

1 ○○○○○○○○
2 ○○○○○○○○
3 ○○○○○○○○
4 ○○○○○○○○
5 ○○○○○○○○
6 ○○○○○○○○
7 ○○○○○○○○
8 ○○○○○○○○
9 ○○○○○○○○
10 ○○○○○○○○
11 ○○○○○○○○
12 ○○○○○○○○
13 ○○○○○○○○
14 ○○○○○○○○
15 ○○○○○○○○

16 ○○○○○○○○
17 ○○○○○○○○
18 ○○○○○○○○
19 ○○○○○○○○
20 ○○○○○○○○
21 ○○○○○○○○
22 ○○○○○○○○
23 ○○○○○○○○
24 ○○○○○○○○
25 ○○○○○○○○
26 ○○○○○○○○
27 ○○○○○○○○
28 ○○○○○○○○
29 ○○○○○○○○

# Alcohol Tracker

One glass = one unit (recommended weekly intake: no more than 14 units)

Single shot of spirits (25 ml) = 1 unit
Alcopop (275 ml) = 1.5 units
Small glass of wine (125 ml) = 1.5 units
Pint of lower-strength lager/beer/cider
(ABV 3.6%) = 2 units

Standard glass of wine (175 ml) = 2.1 units
Pint of higher-strength lager/beer/cider
(ABV 5.2%) = 3 units
Large glass of wine (250 ml) = 3 units

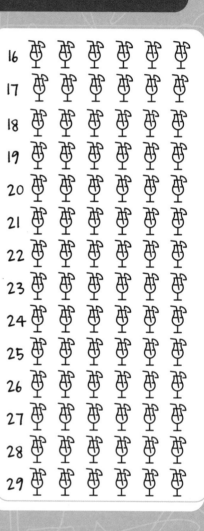

1
2
3
4
5
6
7
8
9
10
11
12
13
14
15
16
17
18
19
20
21
22
23
24
25
26
27
28
29

# Wellness Tracker

On each day this month, colour in one
shape according to how you feel.

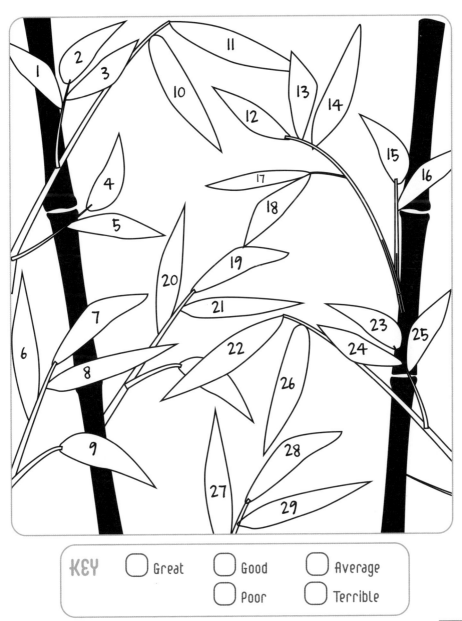

KEY
- ⭘ Great
- ⭘ Good
- ⭘ Average
- ⭘ Poor
- ⭘ Terrible

The groundwork
for all happiness
is good health.

LEIGH HUNT

# TOP TIPS

## SETTING GOALS

When it comes to fitness, everybody's goals are a little different. They all share one similarity though: they help you stay motivated. Without goals, it's too easy to skip a session, a match or a run because you're not aiming for anything. Similarly, if you set huge, unrealistic goals, it's easy to get demotivated and overwhelmed.

So, how do you make goals that work for you? You make them SMART. SMART is an acronym that stands for Specific, Measurable, Attainable, Relevant and Time-Bound, and goals that meet these criteria tend to be easier to stick with. Here's an example for the goal of running a parkrun.

**S**pecific: Take part in a parkrun event

**M**easurable: I will have completed the goal when the event is done

**A**ttainable: The 5k distance is realistic for my fitness level

**R**elevant: It will build my fitness and confidence

**T**ime-bound: I will partake in the event this month

# Exercise Tracker

Using the key, colour in and add patterns to the trainers in the
space below to help you gauge how much exercise you're doing.
If you feel like you're smashing it, then keep up the good work.
But if you think you could do better, there's always next month!

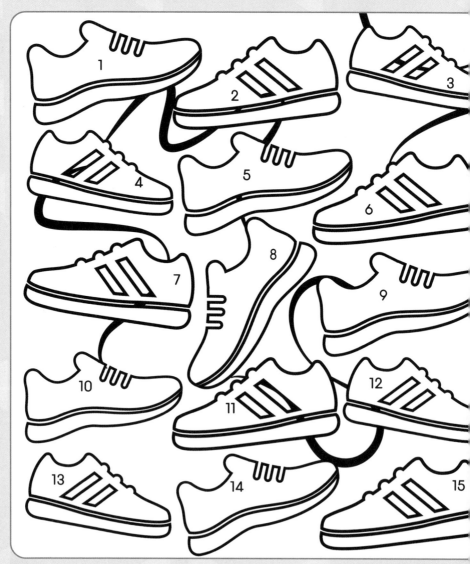

# KEY

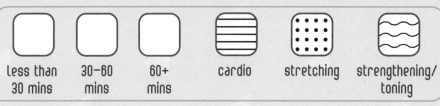

less than 30 mins | 30–60 mins | 60+ mins | cardio | stretching | strengthening/toning

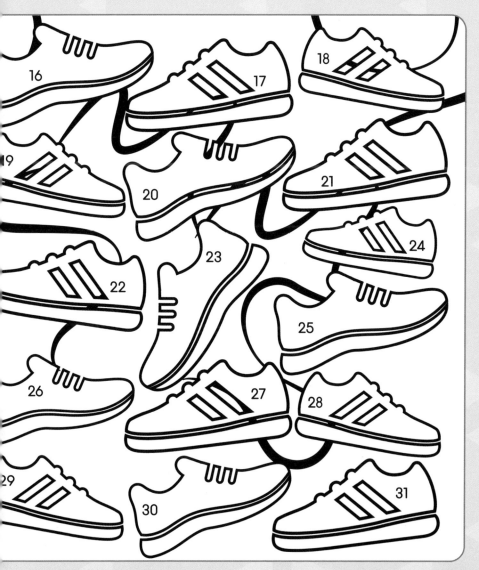

16

17

18

19

20

21

22

23

24

25

26

27

28

29

30

31

I RESPECT MY BODY BECAUSE MY BODY DESERVES RESPECT

## HYDRATION HACKS

Considering that humans made the journey from cave dwellers to astronauts, it's surprising that we often find ourselves fairly bad at doing one of the most important things for survival: drinking water.

Water is essential for the running of your body; even bones are almost a third water. It only takes a slight drop in supply for your body and brain to operate on a sub-optimal level. Lack of focus, impaired physical performance and dull skin are just a few symptoms.

Here are some tips to help you drink enough water:

- Start your day with a glass of water

- Carry a refillable water bottle with you and keep it in sight and within reach

- Set a reminder to drink, particularly a good hour before a workout

- Anchor it to another habit, such as going to the bathroom or making a coffee

# Five-a-Day Tracker

Each apple = one of your five fruits or vegetables a day

| | |
|---|---|
| 1 | 16 |
| 2 | 17 |
| 3 | 18 |
| 4 | 19 |
| 5 | 20 |
| 6 | 21 |
| 7 | 22 |
| 8 | 23 |
| 9 | 24 |
| 10 | 25 |
| 11 | 26 |
| 12 | 27 |
| 13 | 28 |
| 14 | 29 |
| 15 | 30 |
| | 31 |

# My Goals and Achievements

Don't worry if you don't manage to achieve your goals —
any progress is great and there's always next month!

## My goal(s) for this month

Example goal: Drink eight glasses of water a day

- ................................................... **ACHIEVED Y/N**

- ................................................... **ACHIEVED Y/N**

- ................................................... **ACHIEVED Y/N**

## Steps to make the goal(s) achievable

Example steps: Write down my reasons for being hydrated;
make drinking water part of certain activities, such as
eating meals; set alarms to remind myself to drink

- ...................................................

  ...................................................

- ...................................................

  ...................................................

- ...................................................

  ...................................................

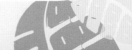

# Healthy Weight Tracker

Keeping track of your weight doesn't need to fill you with dread as long as you remind yourself that the figures that appear on the scales are just one part of your healthy body maintenance. Weight fluctuations occur throughout the day and can be caused by many factors including hormone levels, so don't worry about small increases or decreases. The most important information you want to keep track of is your BMI, as this shows you whether you are a healthy weight for your height.

Try to weigh yourself on the same day at the same time each week.

Don't scrutinize the small numbers; maintaining a healthy lifestyle is what's most important.

|        | Week One | Week Two | Week Three | Week Four |
|--------|----------|----------|------------|-----------|
| Weight |          |          |            |           |
| BMI    |          |          |            |           |
| Chest  |          |          |            |           |
| Waist  |          |          |            |           |
| Hips   |          |          |            |           |

To work out your BMI, calculate your weight divided by your height squared (in metric). Find the BMI chart on page 152 to see the results of your BMI.

# Water Tracker

One drop = one glass (400 ml)

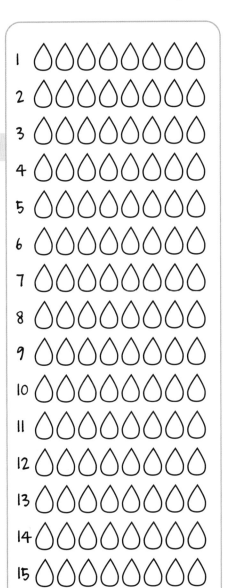

# Alcohol Tracker

One glass = one unit (recommended weekly intake: no more than 14 units)

Single shot of spirits (25 ml) = 1 unit
Alcopop (275 ml) = 1.5 units
Small glass of wine (125 ml) = 1.5 units
Pint of lower-strength lager/beer/cider
(ABV 3.6%) = 2 units

Standard glass of wine (175 ml) = 2.1 units
Pint of higher-strength lager/beer/cider
(ABV 5.2%) = 3 units
Large glass of wine (250 ml) = 3 units

1
2
3
4
5
6
7
8
9
10
11
12
13
14
15
16

17
18
19
20
21
22
23
24
25
26
27
28
29
30
31

# Wellness Tracker

On each day this month, colour in one
shape according to how you feel.

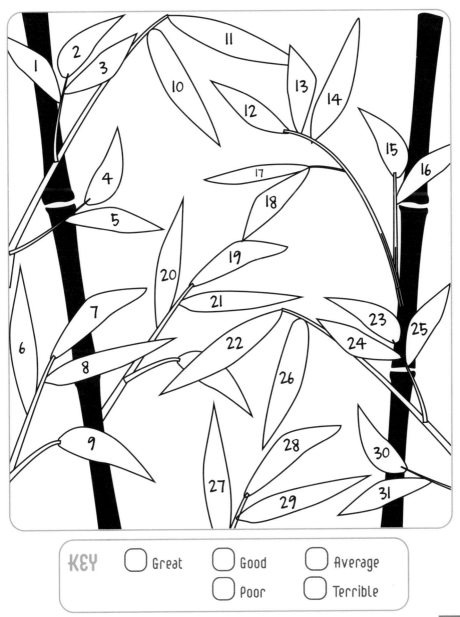

**KEY**

- ◯ Great
- ◯ Good
- ◯ Average
- ◯ Poor
- ◯ Terrible

Don't use scepticism
as a thinly veiled
excuse for inaction
or remaining in
your comfort zone.

TIM FERRISS

# TOP TIPS

## CHOOSING FITNESS ACTIVITIES

There are so many fitness classes, sports and active hobbies that choosing one can feel a little overwhelming. However, when you assess your own needs, wants and goals, you can pick activities you're more likely to enjoy and stick with.

Here are some great ways to pick an activity for you:

- **Frugal or funds:** Got other financial priorities? Choose free or ultra-affordable activities. Second-hand sports equipment is a good option if you need to buy gear. If you can allocate some funds, leisure centre memberships can offer a wide range of activities.

- **Get goals:** Want to run a marathon? Endurance activities will help you out. Want to release stress? Try kick-boxing or taekwondo.

- **Be balanced:** The best fitness plan is a varied one, so if you love your high-intensity spinning class, consider adding a calming yoga session into your week and vice versa.

# Exercise Tracker

Using the key, colour in and add patterns to the trainers in the space below to help you gauge how much exercise you're doing. If you feel like you're smashing it, then keep up the good work. But if you think you could do better, there's always next month!

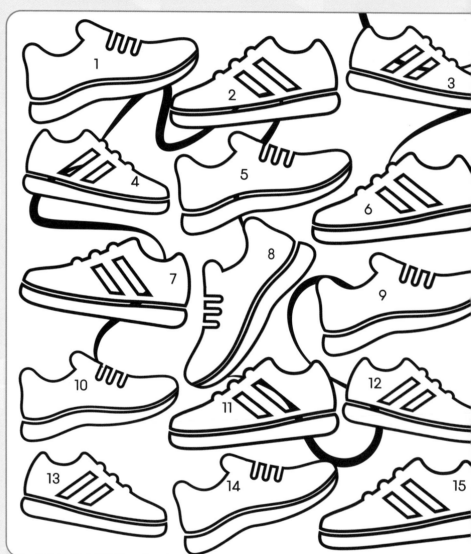

# KEY

 less than 30 mins

 30–60 mins

 60+ mins

 cardio

 stretching

strengthening/ toning

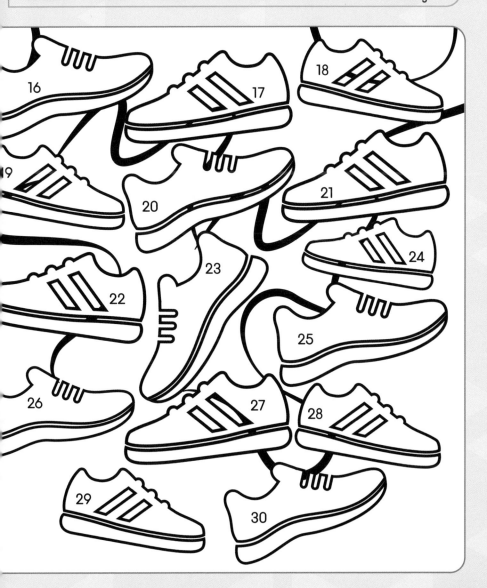

I NOURISH
MY BODY WITH
HEALTHY FOODS
AND MY MIND
WITH HEALTHY
THOUGHTS

# TOP TIPS

## SHOPPING FOR HEALTH

Avoiding the snack aisles can be easier said than done, but two initial rules can help you with healthy, mindful food shopping. The first is probably one you're already familiar with: never shop for food while hungry. The second is to make a list and stick to it.

Here are some more easy ways to fill your shopping basket with food that'll make you feel your best:

- **Buy the rainbow:** Stock up on vegetables of as many different colours as possible because they're packed with different nutrients, antioxidants and flavour.

- **Swap white for brown:** Choose brown or wholemeal rice, pasta and flour to get extra fibre, vitamins and minerals.

- **Beeline for beans:** Chock full of protein, fibre and minerals, beans are versatile and fantastic for your health.

- **DIY snacks:** Oats, nuts and seeds are the core components for making your own delicious snack bars. Add in something sweet like dried dates and skip added sugar entirely.

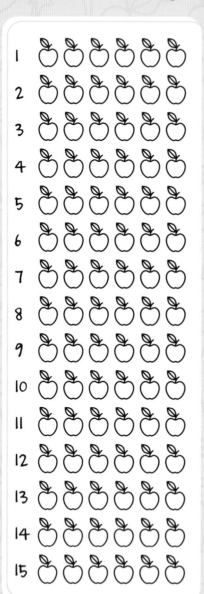

# Five-a-Day Tracker

Each apple = one of your five fruits or vegetables a day

| | | | | | | |
|---|---|---|---|---|---|---|
| 1 | 🍎 | 🍎 | 🍎 | 🍎 | 🍎 | 🍎 |
| 2 | 🍎 | 🍎 | 🍎 | 🍎 | 🍎 | 🍎 |
| 3 | 🍎 | 🍎 | 🍎 | 🍎 | 🍎 | 🍎 |
| 4 | 🍎 | 🍎 | 🍎 | 🍎 | 🍎 | 🍎 |
| 5 | 🍎 | 🍎 | 🍎 | 🍎 | 🍎 | 🍎 |
| 6 | 🍎 | 🍎 | 🍎 | 🍎 | 🍎 | 🍎 |
| 7 | 🍎 | 🍎 | 🍎 | 🍎 | 🍎 | 🍎 |
| 8 | 🍎 | 🍎 | 🍎 | 🍎 | 🍎 | 🍎 |
| 9 | 🍎 | 🍎 | 🍎 | 🍎 | 🍎 | 🍎 |
| 10 | 🍎 | 🍎 | 🍎 | 🍎 | 🍎 | 🍎 |
| 11 | 🍎 | 🍎 | 🍎 | 🍎 | 🍎 | 🍎 |
| 12 | 🍎 | 🍎 | 🍎 | 🍎 | 🍎 | 🍎 |
| 13 | 🍎 | 🍎 | 🍎 | 🍎 | 🍎 | 🍎 |
| 14 | 🍎 | 🍎 | 🍎 | 🍎 | 🍎 | 🍎 |
| 15 | 🍎 | 🍎 | 🍎 | 🍎 | 🍎 | 🍎 |
| 16 | 🍎 | 🍎 | 🍎 | 🍎 | 🍎 | 🍎 |
| 17 | 🍎 | 🍎 | 🍎 | 🍎 | 🍎 | 🍎 |
| 18 | 🍎 | 🍎 | 🍎 | 🍎 | 🍎 | 🍎 |
| 19 | 🍎 | 🍎 | 🍎 | 🍎 | 🍎 | 🍎 |
| 20 | 🍎 | 🍎 | 🍎 | 🍎 | 🍎 | 🍎 |
| 21 | 🍎 | 🍎 | 🍎 | 🍎 | 🍎 | 🍎 |
| 22 | 🍎 | 🍎 | 🍎 | 🍎 | 🍎 | 🍎 |
| 23 | 🍎 | 🍎 | 🍎 | 🍎 | 🍎 | 🍎 |
| 24 | 🍎 | 🍎 | 🍎 | 🍎 | 🍎 | 🍎 |
| 25 | 🍎 | 🍎 | 🍎 | 🍎 | 🍎 | 🍎 |
| 26 | 🍎 | 🍎 | 🍎 | 🍎 | 🍎 | 🍎 |
| 27 | 🍎 | 🍎 | 🍎 | 🍎 | 🍎 | 🍎 |
| 28 | 🍎 | 🍎 | 🍎 | 🍎 | 🍎 | 🍎 |
| 29 | 🍎 | 🍎 | 🍎 | 🍎 | 🍎 | 🍎 |
| 30 | 🍎 | 🍎 | 🍎 | 🍎 | 🍎 | 🍎 |

# My Goals and Achievements

Don't worry if you don't manage to achieve your goals —
any progress is great and there's always next month!

## My goal(s) for this month

Example goal: Make myself lunch every working day

- ..................................................... **ACHIEVED Y/N**

- ..................................................... **ACHIEVED Y/N**

- ..................................................... **ACHIEVED Y/N**

## Steps to make the goal(s) achievable

Example steps: Write a short list of healthy lunch ideas;
each week, buy the exact ingredients I need;
prep as much as I can the evening before

- .....................................................
  .....................................................

- .....................................................
  .....................................................

- .....................................................
  .....................................................

# Healthy Weight Tracker

Keeping track of your weight doesn't need to fill you with dread as long as you remind yourself that the figures that appear on the scales are just one part of your healthy body maintenance. Weight fluctuations occur throughout the day and can be caused by many factors including hormone levels, so don't worry about small increases or decreases. The most important information you want to keep track of is your BMI, as this shows you whether you are a healthy weight for your height.

Try to weigh yourself on the same day at the same time each week.

Don't scrutinize the small numbers; maintaining a healthy lifestyle is what's most important.

|  | Week One | Week Two | Week Three | Week four |
|---|---|---|---|---|
| Weight |  |  |  |  |
| BMI |  |  |  |  |
| Chest |  |  |  |  |
| Waist |  |  |  |  |
| Hips |  |  |  |  |

To work out your BMI, calculate your weight divided by your height squared (in metric). Find the BMI chart on page 152 to see the results of your BMI.

# Water Tracker

One drop = one glass (400 ml)

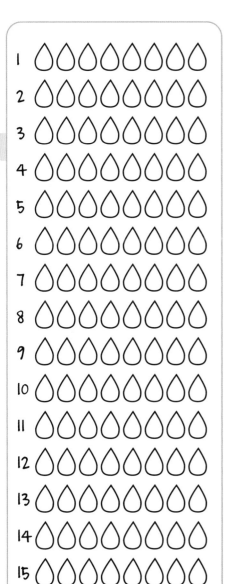

1 ⬦⬦⬦⬦⬦⬦⬦⬦
2 ⬦⬦⬦⬦⬦⬦⬦⬦
3 ⬦⬦⬦⬦⬦⬦⬦⬦
4 ⬦⬦⬦⬦⬦⬦⬦⬦
5 ⬦⬦⬦⬦⬦⬦⬦⬦
6 ⬦⬦⬦⬦⬦⬦⬦⬦
7 ⬦⬦⬦⬦⬦⬦⬦⬦
8 ⬦⬦⬦⬦⬦⬦⬦⬦
9 ⬦⬦⬦⬦⬦⬦⬦⬦
10 ⬦⬦⬦⬦⬦⬦⬦⬦
11 ⬦⬦⬦⬦⬦⬦⬦⬦
12 ⬦⬦⬦⬦⬦⬦⬦⬦
13 ⬦⬦⬦⬦⬦⬦⬦⬦
14 ⬦⬦⬦⬦⬦⬦⬦⬦
15 ⬦⬦⬦⬦⬦⬦⬦⬦

16 ⬦⬦⬦⬦⬦⬦⬦⬦
17 ⬦⬦⬦⬦⬦⬦⬦⬦
18 ⬦⬦⬦⬦⬦⬦⬦⬦
19 ⬦⬦⬦⬦⬦⬦⬦⬦
20 ⬦⬦⬦⬦⬦⬦⬦⬦
21 ⬦⬦⬦⬦⬦⬦⬦⬦
22 ⬦⬦⬦⬦⬦⬦⬦⬦
23 ⬦⬦⬦⬦⬦⬦⬦⬦
24 ⬦⬦⬦⬦⬦⬦⬦⬦
25 ⬦⬦⬦⬦⬦⬦⬦⬦
26 ⬦⬦⬦⬦⬦⬦⬦⬦
27 ⬦⬦⬦⬦⬦⬦⬦⬦
28 ⬦⬦⬦⬦⬦⬦⬦⬦
29 ⬦⬦⬦⬦⬦⬦⬦⬦
30 ⬦⬦⬦⬦⬦⬦⬦⬦

# Alcohol Tracker

One glass = one unit (recommended weekly intake: no more than 14 units)

Single shot of spirits (25 ml) = 1 unit
Alcopop (275 ml) = 1.5 units
Small glass of wine (125 ml) = 1.5 units
Pint of lower-strength lager/beer/cider
(ABV 3.6%) = 2 units

Standard glass of wine (175 ml) = 2.1 units
Pint of higher-strength lager/beer/cider
(ABV 5.2%) = 3 units
Large glass of wine (250 ml) = 3 units

| | | | | | |
|---|---|---|---|---|---|
| 1 | | | | | |
| 2 | | | | | |
| 3 | | | | | |
| 4 | | | | | |
| 5 | | | | | |
| 6 | | | | | |
| 7 | | | | | |
| 8 | | | | | |
| 9 | | | | | |
| 10 | | | | | |
| 11 | | | | | |
| 12 | | | | | |
| 13 | | | | | |
| 14 | | | | | |
| 15 | | | | | |
| 16 | | | | | |
| 17 | | | | | |
| 18 | | | | | |
| 19 | | | | | |
| 20 | | | | | |
| 21 | | | | | |
| 22 | | | | | |
| 23 | | | | | |
| 24 | | | | | |
| 25 | | | | | |
| 26 | | | | | |
| 27 | | | | | |
| 28 | | | | | |
| 29 | | | | | |
| 30 | | | | | |

# Wellness Tracker

On each day this month, colour in one
shape according to how you feel.

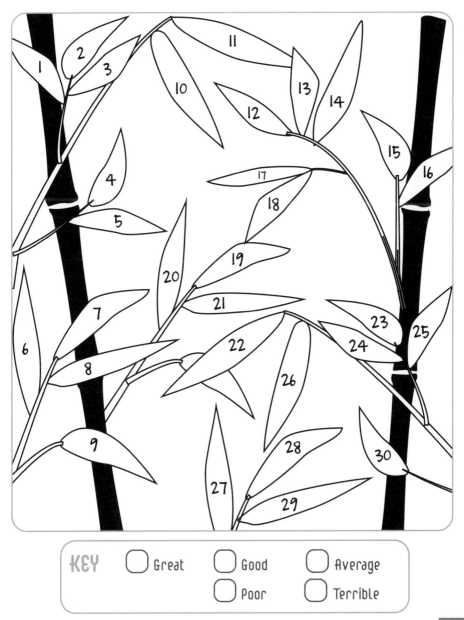

KEY  ◯ Great  ◯ Good  ◯ Average
                ◯ Poor  ◯ Terrible

Failure I can
live with. Not
trying is what
I can't handle.

SANYA RICHARDS-ROSS

# TOP TIPS

## SNACK ON HEALTH

Everywhere you look in supermarkets, coffee shops and even gyms, snacks are within easy reach. These between-meal foods satisfy an immediate urge, but we often don't realize how much extra salt, sugar and saturated fat we're adding into our daily diet.

There are two steps to healthy snacking. Firstly, consider whether you're hungry at all. It's easy to reach for snacks when you're bored, thirsty, emotional or in a place that encourages it, like a cinema. That "hunger" might be sated by drinking water or simply doing something else. Secondly, if you do need a little fuel boost, do just that: opt for something that will fuel you with good nutrients that provide what you need.

Some healthy snack ideas include:

- Bananas, apples and other fruits

- Nuts without additives (no sugar-coating here!)

- Wholewheat toast or crackers

- Vegetable sticks with dips like hummus or guacamole

# Exercise Tracker

Using the key, colour in and add patterns to the trainers in the space below to help you gauge how much exercise you're doing. If you feel like you're smashing it, then keep up the good work. But if you think you could do better, there's always next month!

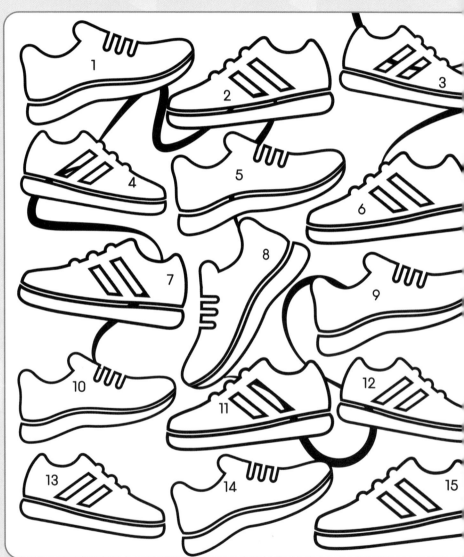

# KEY

 less than 30 mins

 30–60 mins

 60+ mins

 cardio

 stretching

 strengthening/ toning

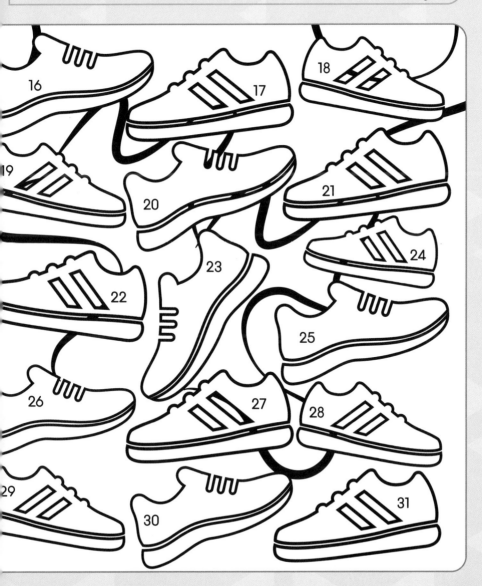

I GIVE MYSELF
PERMISSION TO
SHAKE IT OUT, DANCE
AND CELEBRATE
MY BODY

# TOP TIPS

## GETTING BENDY

While the word "flexibility" might conjure images of yogis in the splits, everyday flexibility is far more straightforward, and important, than that. An inflexible body is more prone to injury than a flexible one, and any injury can derail your fitness journey faster than you can say "ice pack please". When your flexibility is good, you have a wider and more supported range of motion, and your muscles and tendons can take more impact without damage.

Here are a few ideas to get you started on the path to great flexibility.

- Incorporate a yoga session once or twice a week

- Warm up and warm down after any workout

- Do a morning stretch routine every day, such as a yogic sun salutation

- Ensure you stay hydrated

- Pick some desk stretches to do throughout the day at work

- Join a flexibility and conditioning class

# Five-a-Day Tracker

### Each apple = one of your five fruits or vegetables a day

| | | |
|---|---|---|
| 1  🍎🍎🍎🍎🍎🍎 | 16 🍎🍎🍎🍎🍎🍎 |
| 2  🍎🍎🍎🍎🍎🍎 | 17 🍎🍎🍎🍎🍎🍎 |
| 3  🍎🍎🍎🍎🍎🍎 | 18 🍎🍎🍎🍎🍎🍎 |
| 4  🍎🍎🍎🍎🍎🍎 | 19 🍎🍎🍎🍎🍎🍎 |
| 5  🍎🍎🍎🍎🍎🍎 | 20 🍎🍎🍎🍎🍎🍎 |
| 6  🍎🍎🍎🍎🍎🍎 | 21 🍎🍎🍎🍎🍎🍎 |
| 7  🍎🍎🍎🍎🍎🍎 | 22 🍎🍎🍎🍎🍎🍎 |
| 8  🍎🍎🍎🍎🍎🍎 | 23 🍎🍎🍎🍎🍎🍎 |
| 9  🍎🍎🍎🍎🍎🍎 | 24 🍎🍎🍎🍎🍎🍎 |
| 10 🍎🍎🍎🍎🍎🍎 | 25 🍎🍎🍎🍎🍎🍎 |
| 11 🍎🍎🍎🍎🍎🍎 | 26 🍎🍎🍎🍎🍎🍎 |
| 12 🍎🍎🍎🍎🍎🍎 | 27 🍎🍎🍎🍎🍎🍎 |
| 13 🍎🍎🍎🍎🍎🍎 | 28 🍎🍎🍎🍎🍎🍎 |
| 14 🍎🍎🍎🍎🍎🍎 | 29 🍎🍎🍎🍎🍎🍎 |
| 15 🍎🍎🍎🍎🍎🍎 | 30 🍎🍎🍎🍎🍎🍎 |
| | 31 🍎🍎🍎🍎🍎🍎 |

# My Goals and Achievements

Don't worry if you don't manage to achieve your goals —
any progress is great and there's always next month!

## My goal(s) for this month

Example goal: Hit 10,000 steps on four days
out of every seven

ACHIEVED
**Y/N**

• .................................................... ACHIEVED **Y/N**

• .................................................... ACHIEVED **Y/N**

• ....................................................

## Steps to make the goal(s) achievable

Example steps: Ensure I have a step counter on my
phone or watch; take the stairs instead of the lift;
walk for short journeys instead of driving

• ....................................................

.....................................................

• ....................................................

.....................................................

• ....................................................

.....................................................

# Healthy Weight Tracker

Keeping track of your weight doesn't need to fill you with dread as long as you remind yourself that the figures that appear on the scales are just one part of your healthy body maintenance. Weight fluctuations occur throughout the day and can be caused by many factors including hormone levels, so don't worry about small increases or decreases. The most important information you want to keep track of is your BMI, as this shows you whether you are a healthy weight for your height.

Try to weigh yourself on the same day at the same time each week.

Don't scrutinize the small numbers; maintaining a healthy lifestyle is what's most important.

|        | Week One | Week Two | Week Three | Week Four |
|--------|----------|----------|------------|-----------|
| Weight |          |          |            |           |
| BMI    |          |          |            |           |
| Chest  |          |          |            |           |
| Waist  |          |          |            |           |
| Hips   |          |          |            |           |

To work out your BMI, calculate your weight divided by your height squared (in metric). Find the BMI chart on page 152 to see the results of your BMI.

# Water Tracker

One drop = one glass (400 ml)

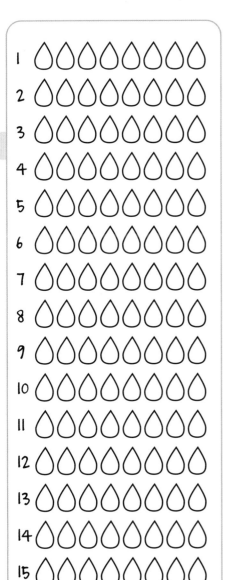

1 ⬭⬭⬭⬭⬭⬭⬭⬭
2 ⬭⬭⬭⬭⬭⬭⬭⬭
3 ⬭⬭⬭⬭⬭⬭⬭⬭
4 ⬭⬭⬭⬭⬭⬭⬭⬭
5 ⬭⬭⬭⬭⬭⬭⬭⬭
6 ⬭⬭⬭⬭⬭⬭⬭⬭
7 ⬭⬭⬭⬭⬭⬭⬭⬭
8 ⬭⬭⬭⬭⬭⬭⬭⬭
9 ⬭⬭⬭⬭⬭⬭⬭⬭
10 ⬭⬭⬭⬭⬭⬭⬭⬭
11 ⬭⬭⬭⬭⬭⬭⬭⬭
12 ⬭⬭⬭⬭⬭⬭⬭⬭
13 ⬭⬭⬭⬭⬭⬭⬭⬭
14 ⬭⬭⬭⬭⬭⬭⬭⬭
15 ⬭⬭⬭⬭⬭⬭⬭⬭

16 ⬭⬭⬭⬭⬭⬭⬭⬭
17 ⬭⬭⬭⬭⬭⬭⬭⬭
18 ⬭⬭⬭⬭⬭⬭⬭⬭
19 ⬭⬭⬭⬭⬭⬭⬭⬭
20 ⬭⬭⬭⬭⬭⬭⬭⬭
21 ⬭⬭⬭⬭⬭⬭⬭⬭
22 ⬭⬭⬭⬭⬭⬭⬭⬭
23 ⬭⬭⬭⬭⬭⬭⬭⬭
24 ⬭⬭⬭⬭⬭⬭⬭⬭
25 ⬭⬭⬭⬭⬭⬭⬭⬭
26 ⬭⬭⬭⬭⬭⬭⬭⬭
27 ⬭⬭⬭⬭⬭⬭⬭⬭
28 ⬭⬭⬭⬭⬭⬭⬭⬭
29 ⬭⬭⬭⬭⬭⬭⬭⬭
30 ⬭⬭⬭⬭⬭⬭⬭⬭
31 ⬭⬭⬭⬭⬭⬭⬭⬭

# Alcohol Tracker

One glass = one unit (recommended weekly intake: no more than 14 units)

Single shot of spirits (25 ml) = 1 unit
Alcopop (275 ml) = 1.5 units
Small glass of wine (125 ml) = 1.5 units
Pint of lower-strength lager/beer/cider
(ABV 3.6%) = 2 units

Standard glass of wine (175 ml) = 2.1 units
Pint of higher-strength lager/beer/cider
(ABV 5.2%) = 3 units
Large glass of wine (250 ml) = 3 units

# Wellness Tracker

On each day this month, colour in one
shape according to how you feel.

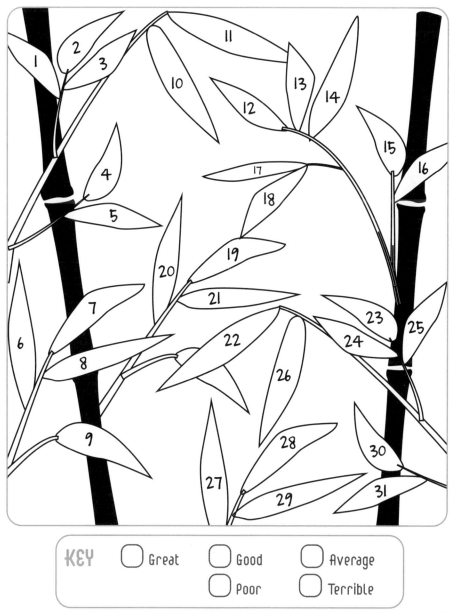

KEY
◯ Great  ◯ Good  ◯ Average
◯ Poor  ◯ Terrible

It was only when I found exercise that I realized the only person I had to prove something to was myself.

JOHN McAVOY

# TOP TIPS

## BUILDING STRENGTH

Building and maintaining strength has many more benefits than simply making moving house a little less tiring. A physically strong body is one you can rely on to protect your joints, support a good posture, and help you balance. This is important at every age but is especially vital in later years when strength prevents falls. Strength also helps you to maintain muscle mass and slows bone density loss.

There are plenty of ways to keep and build strength:

- **Yoga:** Whether online or in a studio, plenty of yoga styles offer full-body strength-building routines.

- **Bodyweight exercises:** With no equipment required, these types of exercises (like push-ups, planks, wall sits and tricep dips) can be done at home at any time.

- **Gym time:** Gyms have plenty of strength-training equipment and knowledgeable staff to help out.

- **Everyday movement:** Walking and cycling as part of your everyday life will naturally build and maintain leg and core strength.

# Exercise Tracker

Using the key, colour in and add patterns to the trainers in the space below to help you gauge how much exercise you're doing. If you feel like you're smashing it, then keep up the good work. But if you think you could do better, there's always next month!

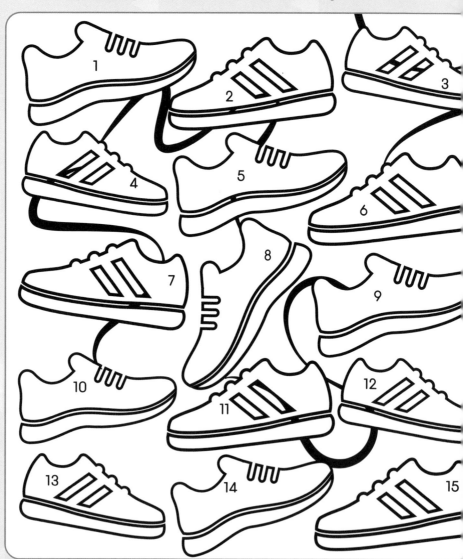

# KEY

| | | | | | |
|---|---|---|---|---|---|
|  |  |  |  | |  |
| less than 30 mins | 30–60 mins | 60+ mins | cardio | stretching | strengthening/ toning |

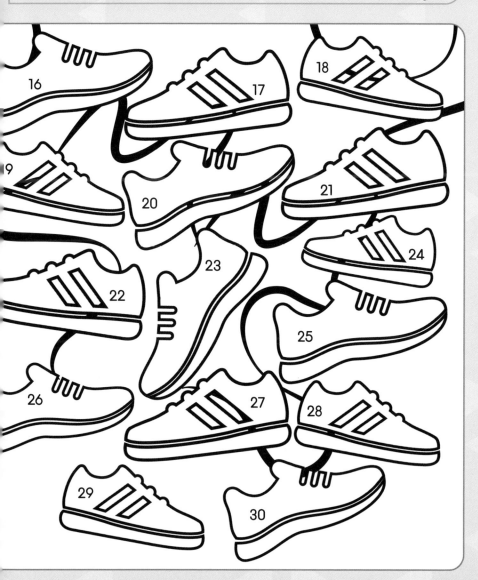

I MAKE
THE CHANGES
I WANT
TO SEE

# TOP TIPS

## REST FOR FITNESS

When you get caught up in a new activity or simply find yourself wanting to work out every day, taking a rest day can feel like wasted time. But in fact, exhausting your body can be just as detrimental as not giving it enough exercise to start with.

Resting is the time when your body can build the muscle it needs and repair any damage done. It's also the time where it replaces its fuel stores burned during your workout and the fluids and electrolytes lost through sweat. Without rest, your body is always playing catch-up until it can't – and at that point you will find yourself truly fatigued.

Rest doesn't mean you have to lie around on the sofa (although that's always fun for a little bit). Restorative yoga, walks and sedate swimming all keep your circulation strong during rest days. Maintaining a healthy diet and drinking plenty of water are important during rest days too.

# Five-a-Day Tracker

Each apple = one of your five fruits or vegetables a day

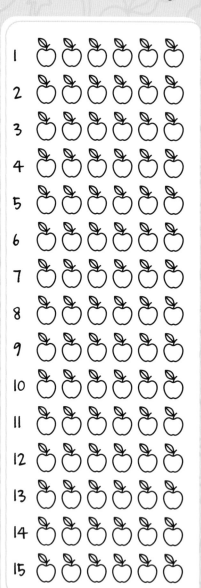

# My Goals and Achievements

Don't worry if you don't manage to achieve your goals —
any progress is great and there's always next month!

## My goal(s) for this month

Example goal: Sleep for 8 hours a night

- .................................................................

ACHIEVED
Y/N

- .................................................................

ACHIEVED
Y/N

- .................................................................

ACHIEVED
Y/N

## Steps to make the goal(s) achievable

Example steps: Set my morning alarm and switch off my
phone an hour before bedtime; read a few pages of a book
each night; go to bed at the same time every night

- .............................................................

.............................................................

- .............................................................

.............................................................

- .............................................................

.............................................................

# Healthy Weight Tracker

Keeping track of your weight doesn't need to fill you with dread as long as you remind yourself that the figures that appear on the scales are just one part of your healthy body maintenance. Weight fluctuations occur throughout the day and can be caused by many factors including hormone levels, so don't worry about small increases or decreases. The most important information you want to keep track of is your BMI, as this shows you whether you are a healthy weight for your height.

Try to weigh yourself on the same day at the same time each week.

Don't scrutinize the small numbers; maintaining a healthy lifestyle is what's most important.

|  | Week One | Week Two | Week Three | Week Four |
|---|---|---|---|---|
| Weight |  |  |  |  |
| BMI |  |  |  |  |
| Chest |  |  |  |  |
| Waist |  |  |  |  |
| Hips |  |  |  |  |

To work out your BMI, calculate your weight divided by your height squared (in metric). Find the BMI chart on page 152 to see the results of your BMI.

# Water Tracker

One drop = one glass (400 ml)

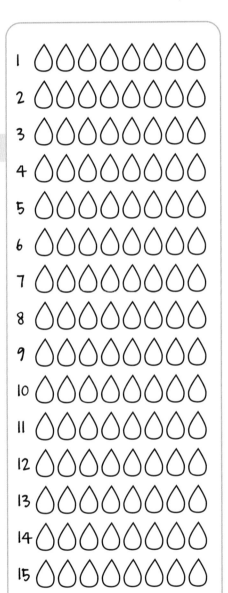

1 ◌◌◌◌◌◌◌◌
2 ◌◌◌◌◌◌◌◌
3 ◌◌◌◌◌◌◌◌
4 ◌◌◌◌◌◌◌◌
5 ◌◌◌◌◌◌◌◌
6 ◌◌◌◌◌◌◌◌
7 ◌◌◌◌◌◌◌◌
8 ◌◌◌◌◌◌◌◌
9 ◌◌◌◌◌◌◌◌
10 ◌◌◌◌◌◌◌◌
11 ◌◌◌◌◌◌◌◌
12 ◌◌◌◌◌◌◌◌
13 ◌◌◌◌◌◌◌◌
14 ◌◌◌◌◌◌◌◌
15 ◌◌◌◌◌◌◌◌

16 ◌◌◌◌◌◌◌◌
17 ◌◌◌◌◌◌◌◌
18 ◌◌◌◌◌◌◌◌
19 ◌◌◌◌◌◌◌◌
20 ◌◌◌◌◌◌◌◌
21 ◌◌◌◌◌◌◌◌
22 ◌◌◌◌◌◌◌◌
23 ◌◌◌◌◌◌◌◌
24 ◌◌◌◌◌◌◌◌
25 ◌◌◌◌◌◌◌◌
26 ◌◌◌◌◌◌◌◌
27 ◌◌◌◌◌◌◌◌
28 ◌◌◌◌◌◌◌◌
29 ◌◌◌◌◌◌◌◌
30 ◌◌◌◌◌◌◌◌

# Alcohol Tracker

One glass = one unit (recommended weekly intake: no more than 14 units)

Single shot of spirits (25 ml) = 1 unit
Alcopop (275 ml) = 1.5 units
Small glass of wine (125 ml) = 1.5 units
Pint of lower-strength lager/beer/cider (ABV 3.6%) = 2 units

Standard glass of wine (175 ml) = 2.1 units
Pint of higher-strength lager/beer/cider (ABV 5.2%) = 3 units
Large glass of wine (250 ml) = 3 units

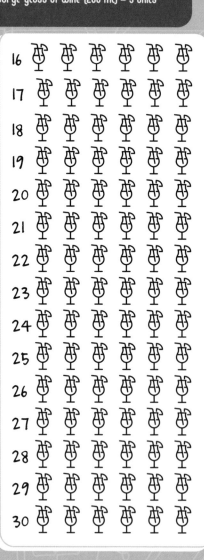

1
2
3
4
5
6
7
8
9
10
11
12
13
14
15

16
17
18
19
20
21
22
23
24
25
26
27
28
29
30

# Wellness Tracker

On each day this month, colour in one
shape according to how you feel.

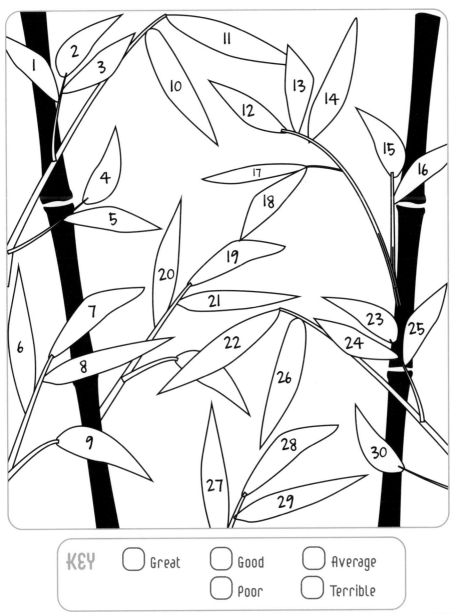

KEY ◯ Great ◯ Good ◯ Average
◯ Poor ◯ Terrible

Sleep is the single most effective thing we can do to reset our brain and body health each day.

MATTHEW WALKER

# TOP TIPS

## SLEEP FOR VICTORY

What's a weekend of bad sleep when you can catch up in the week, right? Wrong. Evidence shows that even mild sleep disruption can contribute to loss of focus, weaken the immune system, slow reaction times and impede learning. Focusing on getting better sleep is one of the best things you can do for your health, fitness and overall well-being. Plus, it's free! Here are some ideas to help you get better quality sleep:

- **Goodbye screens:** Blue light wavelengths, emitted by screens, signal the brain to wake up, so say "no" to electronic screens at least an hour before bed.

- **Hello sun:** Seeing sunlight as soon as you wake up helps set your circadian rhythm and can aid the upcoming night's sleep. Up before the sun? Bright house lights can work too.

- **Caffeine-free:** Consuming caffeine after midday means it's likely to still be in your system come bedtime. Try to avoid caffeine after noon – and watch out for chocolate and green tea, which also contain it.

# Exercise Tracker

Using the key, colour in and add patterns to the trainers in the space below to help you gauge how much exercise you're doing. If you feel like you're smashing it, then keep up the good work. But if you think you could do better, there's always next month!

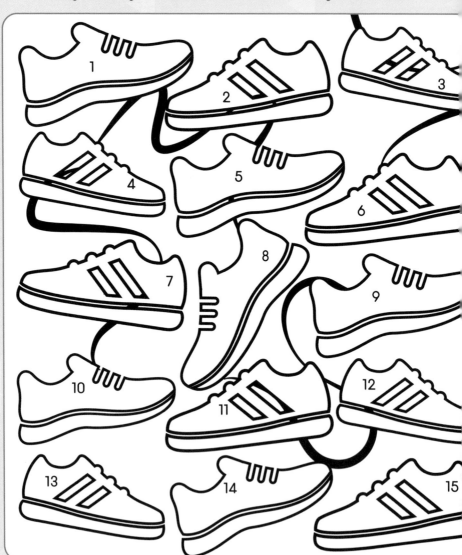

# KEY

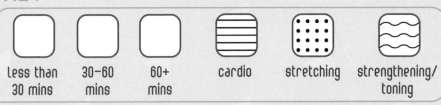

less than 30 mins | 30–60 mins | 60+ mins | cardio | stretching | strengthening/toning

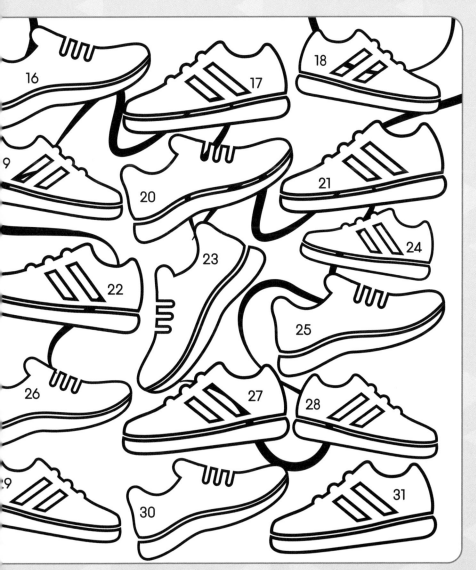

# I HAVE A STRONG AND POWERFUL BODY

## CLUBS AND COMMUNITIES

Exercise is so much more than simply staying trim or getting fit. Many sports have communities that have formed around them, and being able to share your passions with others brings a whole new level to your hobby. This can be hugely motivating, leading you to things you never thought possible. Another great thing about clubs and communities is that they almost always welcome total beginners, and often have a thriving social side too.

From archery and golf clubs to running groups and taekwondo studios, chances are that there are plenty of sports and fitness communities in your area. There's no requirement to be good, and most clubs will have sessions or groups broken up by ability so nobody's left out. If you're not sure where to start, search online for local clubs to see if they have taster sessions. You never know – you might find activities you love and a whole host of new friends too.

# Five-a-Day Tracker

Each apple = one of your five fruits or vegetables a day

| | | |
|---|---|---|
| 1 | 16 |
| 2 | 17 |
| 3 | 18 |
| 4 | 19 |
| 5 | 20 |
| 6 | 21 |
| 7 | 22 |
| 8 | 23 |
| 9 | 24 |
| 10 | 25 |
| 11 | 26 |
| 12 | 27 |
| 13 | 28 |
| 14 | 29 |
| 15 | 30 |
| | 31 |

# My Goals and Achievements

Don't worry if you don't manage to achieve your goals — any progress is great and there's always next month!

## My goal(s) for this month

Example goal: Join a swimming club

- ................................................................

  **ACHIEVED Y/N**

- ................................................................

  **ACHIEVED Y/N**

- ................................................................

  **ACHIEVED Y/N**

## Steps to make the goal(s) achievable

Example steps: Look up local swimming clubs; enquire about a taster session; be open with any members I speak to and ask for any advice I need

- ................................................................

  ................................................................

- ................................................................

  ................................................................

- ................................................................

  ................................................................

# Healthy Weight Tracker

Keeping track of your weight doesn't need to fill you with dread as long as you remind yourself that the figures that appear on the scales are just one part of your healthy body maintenance. Weight fluctuations occur throughout the day and can be caused by many factors including hormone levels, so don't worry about small increases or decreases. The most important information you want to keep track of is your BMI, as this shows you whether you are a healthy weight for your height.

Try to weigh yourself on the same day at the same time each week.

Don't scrutinize the small numbers; maintaining a healthy lifestyle is what's most important.

| | Week One | Week Two | Week Three | Week Four |
|---|---|---|---|---|
| Weight | | | | |
| BMI | | | | |
| Chest | | | | |
| Waist | | | | |
| Hips | | | | |

To work out your BMI, calculate your weight divided by your height squared (in metric). Find the BMI chart on page 152 to see the results of your BMI.

# Water Tracker

One drop = one glass (400 ml)

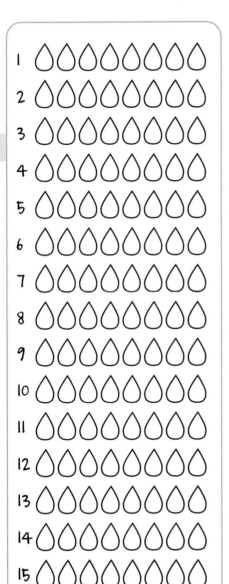

1 ◊◊◊◊◊◊◊◊
2 ◊◊◊◊◊◊◊◊
3 ◊◊◊◊◊◊◊◊
4 ◊◊◊◊◊◊◊◊
5 ◊◊◊◊◊◊◊◊
6 ◊◊◊◊◊◊◊◊
7 ◊◊◊◊◊◊◊◊
8 ◊◊◊◊◊◊◊◊
9 ◊◊◊◊◊◊◊◊
10 ◊◊◊◊◊◊◊◊
11 ◊◊◊◊◊◊◊◊
12 ◊◊◊◊◊◊◊◊
13 ◊◊◊◊◊◊◊◊
14 ◊◊◊◊◊◊◊◊
15 ◊◊◊◊◊◊◊◊

16 ◊◊◊◊◊◊◊◊
17 ◊◊◊◊◊◊◊◊
18 ◊◊◊◊◊◊◊◊
19 ◊◊◊◊◊◊◊◊
20 ◊◊◊◊◊◊◊◊
21 ◊◊◊◊◊◊◊◊
22 ◊◊◊◊◊◊◊◊
23 ◊◊◊◊◊◊◊◊
24 ◊◊◊◊◊◊◊◊
25 ◊◊◊◊◊◊◊◊
26 ◊◊◊◊◊◊◊◊
27 ◊◊◊◊◊◊◊◊
28 ◊◊◊◊◊◊◊◊
29 ◊◊◊◊◊◊◊◊
30 ◊◊◊◊◊◊◊◊
31 ◊◊◊◊◊◊◊◊

# Alcohol Tracker

One glass = one unit (recommended weekly intake: no more than 14 units)

Single shot of spirits (25 ml) = 1 unit
Alcopop (275 ml) = 1.5 units
Small glass of wine (125 ml) = 1.5 units
Pint of lower-strength lager/beer/cider
(ABV 3.6%) = 2 units

Standard glass of wine (175 ml) = 2.1 units
Pint of higher-strength lager/beer/cider
(ABV 5.2%) = 3 units
Large glass of wine (250 ml) = 3 units

| | | | | | | | | | | | | | |
|---|---|---|---|---|---|---|---|---|---|---|---|---|---|
| 1 | | | | | | | 17 | | | | | | |
| 2 | | | | | | | 18 | | | | | | |
| 3 | | | | | | | 19 | | | | | | |
| 4 | | | | | | | 20 | | | | | | |
| 5 | | | | | | | 21 | | | | | | |
| 6 | | | | | | | 22 | | | | | | |
| 7 | | | | | | | 23 | | | | | | |
| 8 | | | | | | | 24 | | | | | | |
| 9 | | | | | | | 25 | | | | | | |
| 10 | | | | | | | 26 | | | | | | |
| 11 | | | | | | | 27 | | | | | | |
| 12 | | | | | | | 28 | | | | | | |
| 13 | | | | | | | 29 | | | | | | |
| 14 | | | | | | | 30 | | | | | | |
| 15 | | | | | | | 31 | | | | | | |
| 16 | | | | | | | | | | | | | |

# Wellness Tracker

On each day this month, colour in one
shape according to how you feel.

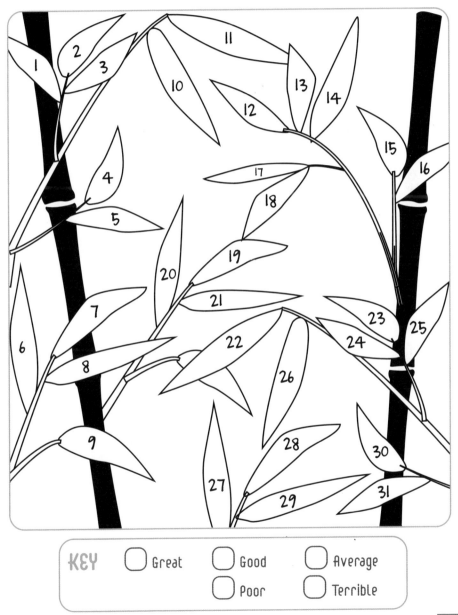

KEY   ◯ Great   ◯ Good   ◯ Average
      ◯ Poor   ◯ Terrible

There is an expression amongst even the most advanced runners that getting your shoes on is the hardest part of any workout.

KATHRINE SWITZER

# TOP TIPS

## HOW TO FALL IN LOVE WITH EXERCISE

Exercise often feels like a chore, but you have the power to flip that. Close your eyes and think about that immense feeling of satisfaction and achievement you get when your workout is done. *That's* what exercise gives you.

No matter how you feel before exercising, take a moment to revel in those memories of strength and empowerment to remind yourself of the great feelings that are coming. All loving relationships take work, and exercise is no different.

After each workout, write a list or say out loud the positive things it made you feel. Such as: this run made me feel like I was flying; I love the feeling of freewheeling down a hill I've cycled up; this Pilates session made me feel connected to myself. By reaffirming the positive things you feel after every workout, it'll be easier to bring that top-of-the-world love into your next one.

# Exercise Tracker

Using the key, colour in and add patterns to the trainers in the space below to help you gauge how much exercise you're doing. If you feel like you're smashing it, then keep up the good work. But if you think you could do better, there's always next month!

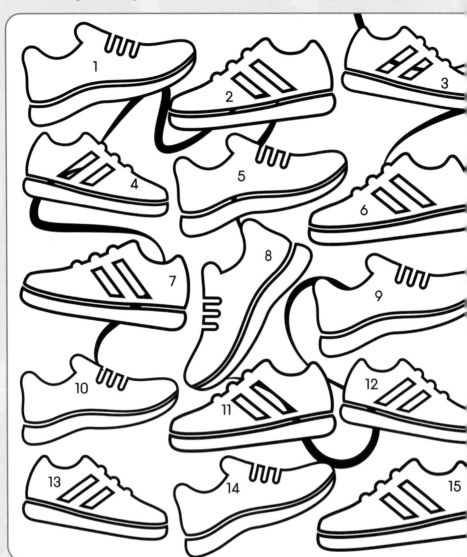

less than 30 mins

 30–60 mins

 60+ mins

 cardio

stretching

strengthening/ toning

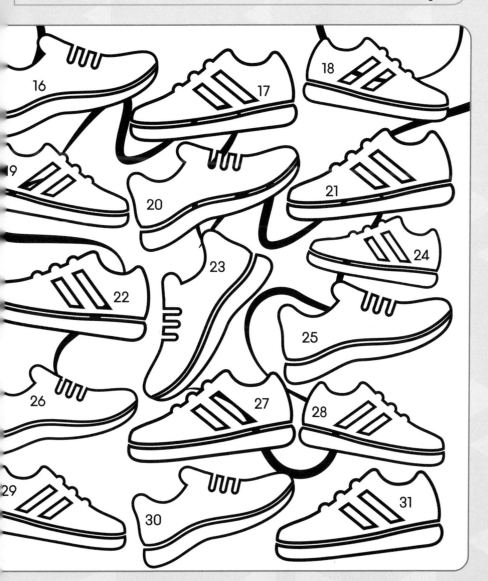

16

17

18

19

20

21

24

23

22

25

26

27

28

29

30

31

# HEALTHY FOOD MAKES ME FEEL ALIVE

# TOP TIPS

## NO LIMITS;
## MORE CHOICES

The idea of giving up chocolate and your favourite type of biscuit isn't exactly fun, and most of us know that the moment we can't have something is the moment we want it the most. So, forget cutting out unhealthy foods from your diet and focus on adding in healthier choices instead. A diet that avoids all sweets, pastries and white pasta can still be unhealthy. However, a diet packed with colourful veg, pulses and legumes with a side of chocolate raisins will be well-balanced.

When you're making your food choices, focus on all the great things you can add in rather than all the foods you should probably be avoiding. When you cook meals based on healthy, wholesome and flavourful ingredients, you're more likely to feel satisfied without reaching for the ice cream afterward.

# Five-a-Day Tracker

Each apple = one of your five fruits or vegetables a day

| | |
|---|---|
| 1 | 🍎🍎🍎🍎🍎🍎 |
| 2 | 🍎🍎🍎🍎🍎🍎 |
| 3 | 🍎🍎🍎🍎🍎🍎 |
| 4 | 🍎🍎🍎🍎🍎🍎 |
| 5 | 🍎🍎🍎🍎🍎🍎 |
| 6 | 🍎🍎🍎🍎🍎🍎 |
| 7 | 🍎🍎🍎🍎🍎🍎 |
| 8 | 🍎🍎🍎🍎🍎🍎 |
| 9 | 🍎🍎🍎🍎🍎🍎 |
| 10 | 🍎🍎🍎🍎🍎🍎 |
| 11 | 🍎🍎🍎🍎🍎🍎 |
| 12 | 🍎🍎🍎🍎🍎🍎 |
| 13 | 🍎🍎🍎🍎🍎🍎 |
| 14 | 🍎🍎🍎🍎🍎🍎 |
| 15 | 🍎🍎🍎🍎🍎🍎 |
| 16 | 🍎🍎🍎🍎🍎🍎 |
| 17 | 🍎🍎🍎🍎🍎🍎 |
| 18 | 🍎🍎🍎🍎🍎🍎 |
| 19 | 🍎🍎🍎🍎🍎🍎 |
| 20 | 🍎🍎🍎🍎🍎🍎 |
| 21 | 🍎🍎🍎🍎🍎🍎 |
| 22 | 🍎🍎🍎🍎🍎🍎 |
| 23 | 🍎🍎🍎🍎🍎🍎 |
| 24 | 🍎🍎🍎🍎🍎🍎 |
| 25 | 🍎🍎🍎🍎🍎🍎 |
| 26 | 🍎🍎🍎🍎🍎🍎 |
| 27 | 🍎🍎🍎🍎🍎🍎 |
| 28 | 🍎🍎🍎🍎🍎🍎 |
| 29 | 🍎🍎🍎🍎🍎🍎 |
| 30 | 🍎🍎🍎🍎🍎🍎 |
| 31 | 🍎🍎🍎🍎🍎🍎 |

# My Goals and Achievements

Don't worry if you don't manage to achieve your goals –
any progress is great and there's always next month!

## My goal(s) for this month

Example goal: Eat my five-a-day

ACHIEVED
Y/N

- .................................................

ACHIEVED
Y/N

- .................................................

ACHIEVED
Y/N

- .................................................

## Steps to make the goal(s) achievable

Example steps: Keep plenty of fruit and vegetables in
the house; plan meals to include at least five portions
across the day (one of fruit, four of veg); find recipes
for green smoothies to give myself a boost

- .................................................
  .................................................

- .................................................
  .................................................

- .................................................
  .................................................

# Healthy Weight Tracker

Keeping track of your weight doesn't need to fill you with dread as long as you remind yourself that the figures that appear on the scales are just one part of your healthy body maintenance. Weight fluctuations occur throughout the day and can be caused by many factors including hormone levels, so don't worry about small increases or decreases. The most important information you want to keep track of is your BMI, as this shows you whether you are a healthy weight for your height.

Try to weigh yourself on the same day at the same time each week.

Don't scrutinize the small numbers; maintaining a healthy lifestyle is what's most important.

|        | Week One | Week Two | Week Three | Week Four |
|--------|----------|----------|------------|-----------|
| Weight |          |          |            |           |
| BMI    |          |          |            |           |
| Chest  |          |          |            |           |
| Waist  |          |          |            |           |
| Hips   |          |          |            |           |

To work out your BMI, calculate your weight divided by your height squared (in metric). Find the BMI chart on page 152 to see the results of your BMI.

# Water Tracker

One drop = one glass (400 ml)

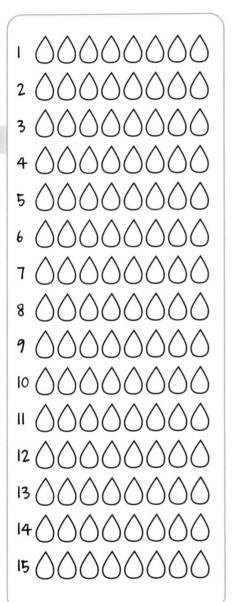

1 ◌◌◌◌◌◌◌◌
2 ◌◌◌◌◌◌◌◌
3 ◌◌◌◌◌◌◌◌
4 ◌◌◌◌◌◌◌◌
5 ◌◌◌◌◌◌◌◌
6 ◌◌◌◌◌◌◌◌
7 ◌◌◌◌◌◌◌◌
8 ◌◌◌◌◌◌◌◌
9 ◌◌◌◌◌◌◌◌
10 ◌◌◌◌◌◌◌◌
11 ◌◌◌◌◌◌◌◌
12 ◌◌◌◌◌◌◌◌
13 ◌◌◌◌◌◌◌◌
14 ◌◌◌◌◌◌◌◌
15 ◌◌◌◌◌◌◌◌

16 ◌◌◌◌◌◌◌◌
17 ◌◌◌◌◌◌◌◌
18 ◌◌◌◌◌◌◌◌
19 ◌◌◌◌◌◌◌◌
20 ◌◌◌◌◌◌◌◌
21 ◌◌◌◌◌◌◌◌
22 ◌◌◌◌◌◌◌◌
23 ◌◌◌◌◌◌◌◌
24 ◌◌◌◌◌◌◌◌
25 ◌◌◌◌◌◌◌◌
26 ◌◌◌◌◌◌◌◌
27 ◌◌◌◌◌◌◌◌
28 ◌◌◌◌◌◌◌◌
29 ◌◌◌◌◌◌◌◌
30 ◌◌◌◌◌◌◌◌
31 ◌◌◌◌◌◌◌◌

# Alcohol Tracker

One glass = one unit (recommended weekly intake: no more than 14 units)

Single shot of spirits (25 ml) = 1 unit
Alcopop (275 ml) = 1.5 units
Small glass of wine (125 ml) = 1.5 units
Pint of lower-strength lager/beer/cider
(ABV 3.6%) = 2 units

Standard glass of wine (175 ml) = 2.1 units
Pint of higher-strength lager/beer/cider
(ABV 5.2%) = 3 units
Large glass of wine (250 ml) = 3 units

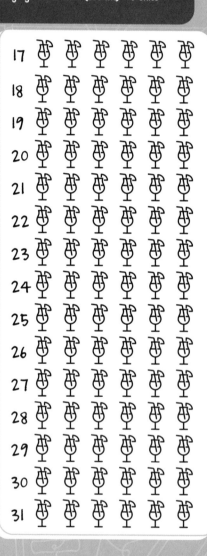

# Wellness Tracker

On each day this month, colour in one
shape according to how you feel.

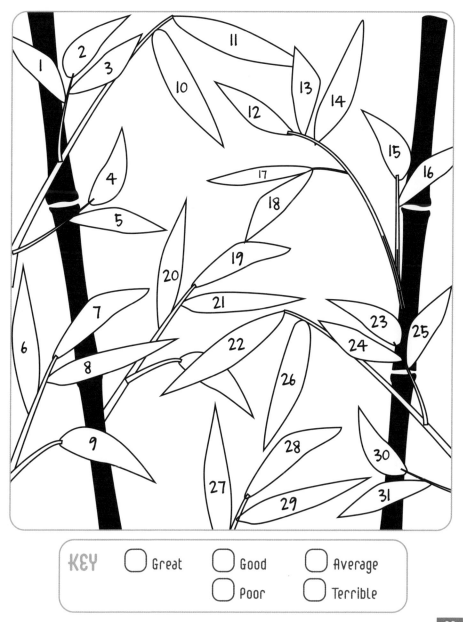

KEY   ◯ Great   ◯ Good   ◯ Average
      ◯ Poor   ◯ Terrible

The only one
who can tell you
"you can't win"
is you, and you
don't have to listen.

JESSICA ENNIS-HILL

# TOP TIPS

## AEROBIC AND ANAEROBIC

The terms "aerobic" and "anaerobic" may sound technical, but they will help you understand your workouts and build a well-rounded routine.

- **Aerobic exercise:** Workouts where your body can take in the amount of oxygen it needs to continue, e.g. normal running, swimming, cycling and dancing

- **Anaerobic exercise:** Workouts that use more oxygen than the body can breathe in, e.g. sprinting, HIIT classes and weightlifting – a.k.a. when you're giving 100 per cent

Your personal fitness level also dictates whether an exercise is one or the other. If you're new to running and try a pace that an experienced runner would find aerobic, you might find yourself quickly running out of breath – so, for you, the workout would be anaerobic. Unless you're deliberately sprinting, this is simply a sign to slow down and build your fitness.

A well-rounded fitness plan includes both types, because aerobic exercise improves cardiovascular function and burns fat while anaerobic exercise builds more muscle, burns fat and strengthens joints.

# Exercise Tracker

Using the key, colour in and add patterns to the trainers in the space below to help you gauge how much exercise you're doing. If you feel like you're smashing it, then keep up the good work. But if you think you could do better, there's always next month!

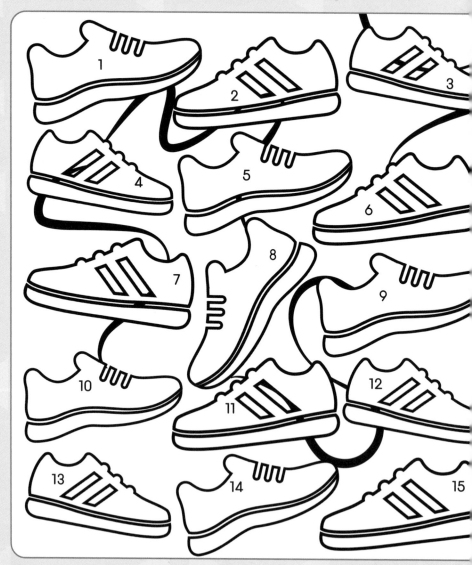

# KEY

| | | | | | |
|---|---|---|---|---|---|
|  |  |  |  |  |  |
| less than 30 mins | 30–60 mins | 60+ mins | cardio | stretching | strengthening/ toning |

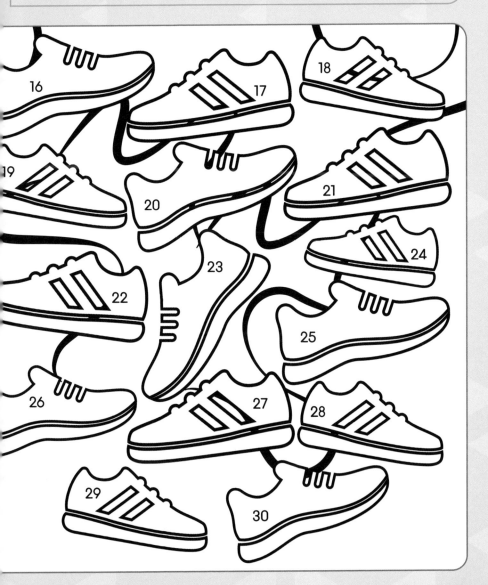

I AM
STRONGER
THAN MY
EXCUSES

# TOP TIPS

## HOW TO REDUCE ALCOHOL INTAKE

Reducing your alcohol intake – or freeing yourself from it entirely – can have a positive effect on your physical and mental health. Alcohol is often high in calories, and can make us crave junk food. In addition, even a small amount can disrupt sleep, cause dehydration and increase anxiety, which has a negative effect overall on our well-being.

The great news is that there are plenty of simple ways to cut back or cut out alcohol. Here are some ideas:

- Choose alcohol-free (and sugar-free) alternatives when you're in a bar

- Suggest non-drinking activities when meeting friends

- Write a short list of reasons why cutting down on alcohol is important to you

- Steer clear of people who encourage you to drink

- Have a couple of reasons you can give, e.g. "I'm doing a no-drinking challenge" or "I want to feel my best tomorrow"

# Five-a-Day Tracker

Each apple = one of your five fruits or vegetables a day

1
2
3
4
5
6
7
8
9
10
11
12
13
14
15

16
17
18
19
20
21
22
23
24
25
26
27
28
29
30

# My Goals and Achievements

Don't worry if you don't manage to achieve your goals —
any progress is great and there's always next month!

## My goal(s) for this month

Example goal: Reduce my alcohol consumption to
two moderate Friday nights drinking a month

ACHIEVED
Y/N

- .................................................................

ACHIEVED
Y/N

- .................................................................

ACHIEVED
Y/N

- .................................................................

## Steps to make the goal(s) achievable

Example steps: Plan my two Fridays, such as dinners with
friends; avoid having alcohol in the house; buy some soft drinks
to keep at home, such as sparkling water or herbal tea

- .................................................................

    .................................................................

- .................................................................

    .................................................................

- .................................................................

    .................................................................

# Healthy Weight Tracker

Keeping track of your weight doesn't need to fill you with dread as long as you remind yourself that the figures that appear on the scales are just one part of your healthy body maintenance. Weight fluctuations occur throughout the day and can be caused by many factors including hormone levels, so don't worry about small increases or decreases. The most important information you want to keep track of is your BMI, as this shows you whether you are a healthy weight for your height.

Try to weigh yourself on the same day at the same time each week.

Don't scrutinize the small numbers; maintaining a healthy lifestyle is what's most important.

|        | Week One | Week Two | Week Three | Week Four |
|--------|----------|----------|------------|-----------|
| Weight |          |          |            |           |
| BMI    |          |          |            |           |
| Chest  |          |          |            |           |
| Waist  |          |          |            |           |
| Hips   |          |          |            |           |

To work out your BMI, calculate your weight divided by your height squared (in metric). Find the BMI chart on page 152 to see the results of your BMI.

# Water Tracker

One drop = one glass (400 ml)

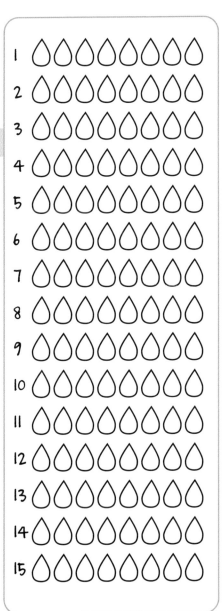

| | |
|---|---|
| 1 ◊◊◊◊◊◊◊◊ | 16 ◊◊◊◊◊◊◊◊ |
| 2 ◊◊◊◊◊◊◊◊ | 17 ◊◊◊◊◊◊◊◊ |
| 3 ◊◊◊◊◊◊◊◊ | 18 ◊◊◊◊◊◊◊◊ |
| 4 ◊◊◊◊◊◊◊◊ | 19 ◊◊◊◊◊◊◊◊ |
| 5 ◊◊◊◊◊◊◊◊ | 20 ◊◊◊◊◊◊◊◊ |
| 6 ◊◊◊◊◊◊◊◊ | 21 ◊◊◊◊◊◊◊◊ |
| 7 ◊◊◊◊◊◊◊◊ | 22 ◊◊◊◊◊◊◊◊ |
| 8 ◊◊◊◊◊◊◊◊ | 23 ◊◊◊◊◊◊◊◊ |
| 9 ◊◊◊◊◊◊◊◊ | 24 ◊◊◊◊◊◊◊◊ |
| 10 ◊◊◊◊◊◊◊◊ | 25 ◊◊◊◊◊◊◊◊ |
| 11 ◊◊◊◊◊◊◊◊ | 26 ◊◊◊◊◊◊◊◊ |
| 12 ◊◊◊◊◊◊◊◊ | 27 ◊◊◊◊◊◊◊◊ |
| 13 ◊◊◊◊◊◊◊◊ | 28 ◊◊◊◊◊◊◊◊ |
| 14 ◊◊◊◊◊◊◊◊ | 29 ◊◊◊◊◊◊◊◊ |
| 15 ◊◊◊◊◊◊◊◊ | 30 ◊◊◊◊◊◊◊◊ |

# Alcohol Tracker

One glass = one unit (recommended weekly intake: no more than 14 units)

Single shot of spirits (25 ml) = 1 unit
Alcopop (275 ml) = 1.5 units
Small glass of wine (125 ml) = 1.5 units
Pint of lower-strength lager/beer/cider
(ABV 3.6%) = 2 units

Standard glass of wine (175 ml) = 2.1 units
Pint of higher-strength lager/beer/cider
(ABV 5.2%) = 3 units
Large glass of wine (250 ml) = 3 units

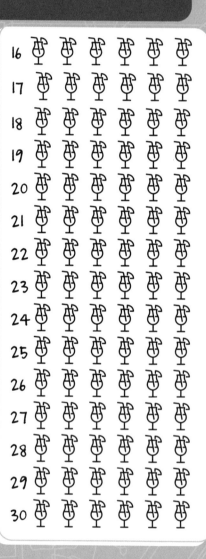

1
2
3
4
5
6
7
8
9
10
11
12
13
14
15

16
17
18
19
20
21
22
23
24
25
26
27
28
29
30

# Wellness Tracker

On each day this month, colour in one
shape according to how you feel.

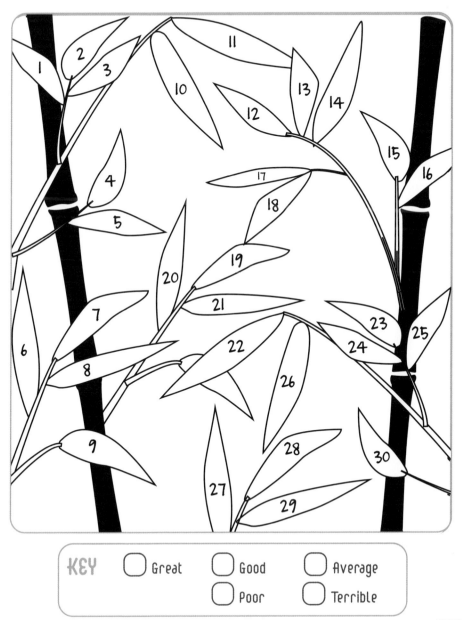

KEY ⬭ Great ⬭ Good ⬭ Average
⬭ Poor ⬭ Terrible

# A healthy outside starts from the inside.

ROBERT URICH

# TOP TIPS

## EXERCISING WHEN YOU'RE BUSY

One of the biggest hurdles to getting fit is finding time to exercise. While you can't create more hours in the day, you can try these tips to create some time, seemingly out of nowhere.

- **Schedule exercise first:** When planning your time, try to schedule fitness sessions as a high priority.

- **Swap for fitness:** Meeting a friend for coffee? Why not suggest a hike, a yoga class or bike ride instead? Got a sunny Sunday with the kids? Playing tag in the park or kicking a football about is great exercise.

- **Prioritize yourself:** It's tempting to prioritize evening emails from your boss, the laundry pile and washing up before yourself, but your health and well-being are simply more important. Carve out pockets of time, even just 15 minutes, for a little exercise every day. As this becomes a habit, you can increase that time and gain confidence in putting your health first.

# Exercise Tracker

Using the key, colour in and add patterns to the trainers in the space below to help you gauge how much exercise you're doing. If you feel like you're smashing it, then keep up the good work. But if you think you could do better, there's always next month!

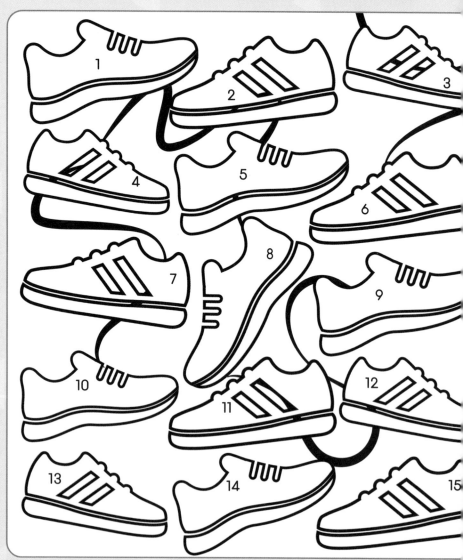

# KEY

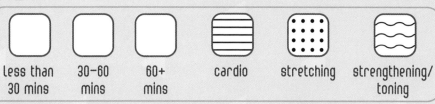

less than 30 mins | 30–60 mins | 60+ mins | cardio | stretching | strengthening/ toning

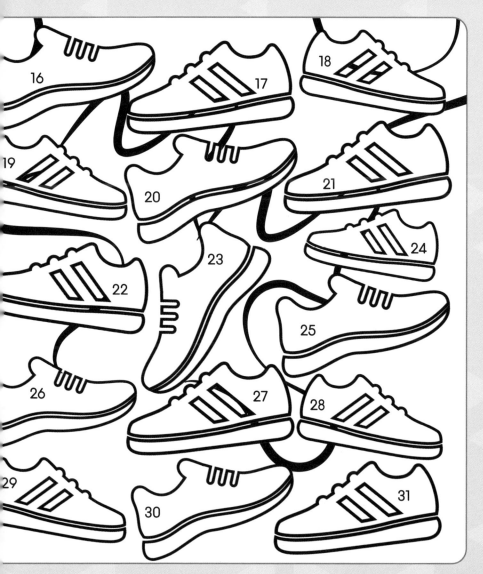

# STRONG BODY = STRONG MIND

# TOP TIPS

## BODY APPRECIATION

Your body is an incredible, complex system. It's a vast network of neurons and a finely tuned structure of muscles that allows you to move about, dance to the radio and cook dinner, all while answering questions from someone else in the room. Everyone's bodies are this fantastic, so why do we struggle so much to appreciate them?

It can be tough to start truly admiring your body, but it's crucial as it'll help you take great care of it, find joy in what it can already do and push it to achieve exciting new challenges.

- **Foster gratitude**: Every day, write down one thing about your body that you're grateful for.

- **Mirror affirmations**: Choose a loving affirmation to say to your body in the mirror every day.

- **Move mindfully**: Five minutes of gentle stretching while focusing on every sensation can generate appreciation for your body's ability.

- **Turn off noise**: Social media making you judge your body? Unfollow those accounts or take a social media break.

# Five-a-Day Tracker

Each apple = one of your five fruits or vegetables a day

| | |
|---|---|
| 1 | 🍎🍎🍎🍎🍎🍎 |
| 2 | 🍎🍎🍎🍎🍎🍎 |
| 3 | 🍎🍎🍎🍎🍎🍎 |
| 4 | 🍎🍎🍎🍎🍎🍎 |
| 5 | 🍎🍎🍎🍎🍎🍎 |
| 6 | 🍎🍎🍎🍎🍎🍎 |
| 7 | 🍎🍎🍎🍎🍎🍎 |
| 8 | 🍎🍎🍎🍎🍎🍎 |
| 9 | 🍎🍎🍎🍎🍎🍎 |
| 10 | 🍎🍎🍎🍎🍎🍎 |
| 11 | 🍎🍎🍎🍎🍎🍎 |
| 12 | 🍎🍎🍎🍎🍎🍎 |
| 13 | 🍎🍎🍎🍎🍎🍎 |
| 14 | 🍎🍎🍎🍎🍎🍎 |
| 15 | 🍎🍎🍎🍎🍎🍎 |
| 16 | 🍎🍎🍎🍎🍎🍎 |
| 17 | 🍎🍎🍎🍎🍎🍎 |
| 18 | 🍎🍎🍎🍎🍎🍎 |
| 19 | 🍎🍎🍎🍎🍎🍎 |
| 20 | 🍎🍎🍎🍎🍎🍎 |
| 21 | 🍎🍎🍎🍎🍎🍎 |
| 22 | 🍎🍎🍎🍎🍎🍎 |
| 23 | 🍎🍎🍎🍎🍎🍎 |
| 24 | 🍎🍎🍎🍎🍎🍎 |
| 25 | 🍎🍎🍎🍎🍎🍎 |
| 26 | 🍎🍎🍎🍎🍎🍎 |
| 27 | 🍎🍎🍎🍎🍎🍎 |
| 28 | 🍎🍎🍎🍎🍎🍎 |
| 29 | 🍎🍎🍎🍎🍎🍎 |
| 30 | 🍎🍎🍎🍎🍎🍎 |
| 31 | 🍎🍎🍎🍎🍎🍎 |

# My Goals and Achievements

Don't worry if you don't manage to achieve your goals —
any progress is great and there's always next month!

## My goal(s) for this month

Example goal: Get 5 cm closer to touching your
toes by the end of the month

ACHIEVED
Y/N

- ....................................................................

ACHIEVED
Y/N

- ....................................................................

ACHIEVED
Y/N

- ....................................................................

## Steps to make the goal(s) achievable

Example steps: Find a few online stretching videos that suit
my goal; learn the types of stretches I need to do; spend 5
minutes each morning and 10 minutes each evening stretching

- ....................................................................

....................................................................

- ....................................................................

....................................................................

- ....................................................................

....................................................................

# Healthy Weight Tracker

Keeping track of your weight doesn't need to fill you with dread as long as you remind yourself that the figures that appear on the scales are just one part of your healthy body maintenance. Weight fluctuations occur throughout the day and can be caused by many factors including hormone levels, so don't worry about small increases or decreases. The most important information you want to keep track of is your BMI, as this shows you whether you are a healthy weight for your height.

Try to weigh yourself on the same day at the same time each week.

Don't scrutinize the small numbers; maintaining a healthy lifestyle is what's most important.

|        | Week One | Week Two | Week Three | Week Four |
|--------|----------|----------|------------|-----------|
| Weight |          |          |            |           |
| BMI    |          |          |            |           |
| Chest  |          |          |            |           |
| Waist  |          |          |            |           |
| Hips   |          |          |            |           |

To work out your BMI, calculate your weight divided by your height squared (in metric). Find the BMI chart on page 152 to see the results of your BMI.

# Water Tracker

One drop = one glass (400 ml)

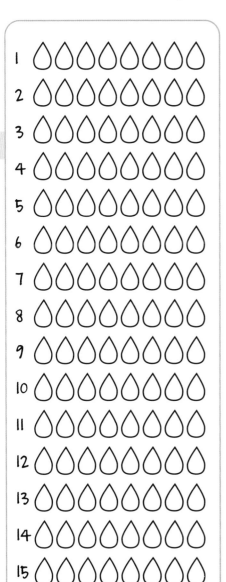

1 ○○○○○○○○
2 ○○○○○○○○
3 ○○○○○○○○
4 ○○○○○○○○
5 ○○○○○○○○
6 ○○○○○○○○
7 ○○○○○○○○
8 ○○○○○○○○
9 ○○○○○○○○
10 ○○○○○○○○
11 ○○○○○○○○
12 ○○○○○○○○
13 ○○○○○○○○
14 ○○○○○○○○
15 ○○○○○○○○

16 ○○○○○○○○
17 ○○○○○○○○
18 ○○○○○○○○
19 ○○○○○○○○
20 ○○○○○○○○
21 ○○○○○○○○
22 ○○○○○○○○
23 ○○○○○○○○
24 ○○○○○○○○
25 ○○○○○○○○
26 ○○○○○○○○
27 ○○○○○○○○
28 ○○○○○○○○
29 ○○○○○○○○
30 ○○○○○○○○
31 ○○○○○○○○

# Alcohol Tracker

One glass = one unit (recommended weekly intake: no more than 14 units)

Single shot of spirits (25 ml) = 1 unit
Alcopop (275 ml) = 1.5 units
Small glass of wine (125 ml) = 1.5 units
Pint of lower-strength lager/beer/cider
(ABV 3.6%) = 2 units

Standard glass of wine (175 ml) = 2.1 units
Pint of higher-strength lager/beer/cider
(ABV 5.2%) = 3 units
Large glass of wine (250 ml) = 3 units

1
2
3
4
5
6
7
8
9
10
11
12
13
14
15
16

17
18
19
20
21
22
23
24
25
26
27
28
29
30
31

# Wellness Tracker

On each day this month, colour in one
shape according to how you feel.

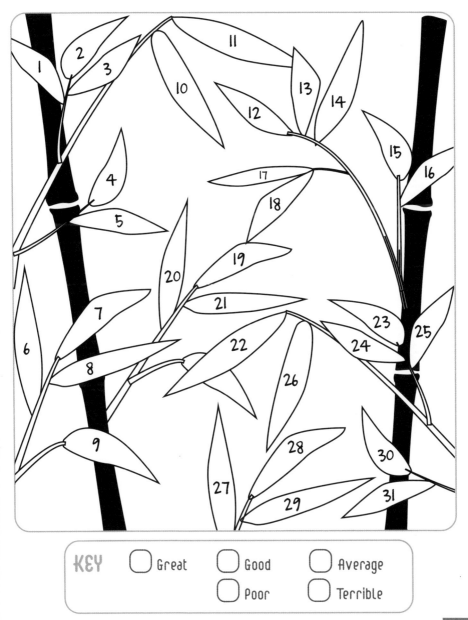

KEY  ◯ Great   ◯ Good   ◯ Average
     ◯ Poor   ◯ Terrible

The first "No"
you hear should
never come
from you.

EVY POUMPOURAS

# TOP TIPS

## ACHE OR INJURY?

On your fitness journey, you'll feel all sorts of niggles and aches that you can't quite put your finger on. The main question is: is this the beginning of an injury or not? Much of the time, it can be tricky to know.

The best cure for sports injuries is prevention. Warming up and down, staying hydrated and fuelled, resting often and building flexibility are all important. With running, cycling, weightlifting and bodyweight exercises, improper form can cause injury, so seek out specialist advice: a personal trainer in the gym, a running gait analyst in a sports store or a bike fit specialist in a cycle shop can all help you get started with the right form and fit.

If you feel a sudden pain, stop what you're doing immediately. It may well turn out to be nothing, but it's far safer to stop than to continue and turn a twinge into a full-blown injury.

# Exercise Tracker

Using the key, colour in and add patterns to the trainers in the space below to help you gauge how much exercise you're doing. If you feel like you're smashing it, then keep up the good work. But if you think you could do better, there's always next month!

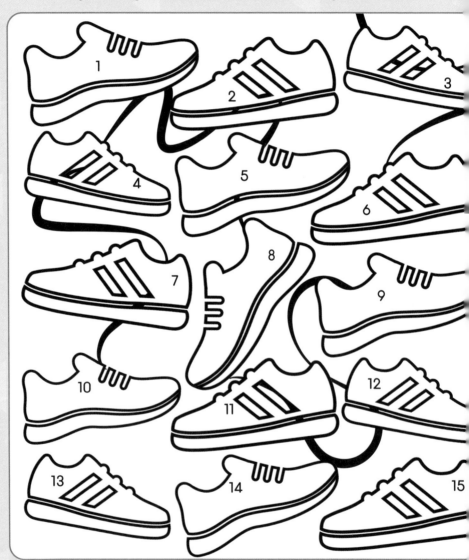

# KEY

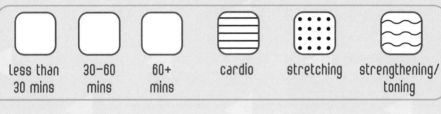

less than 30 mins | 30–60 mins | 60+ mins | cardio | stretching | strengthening/toning

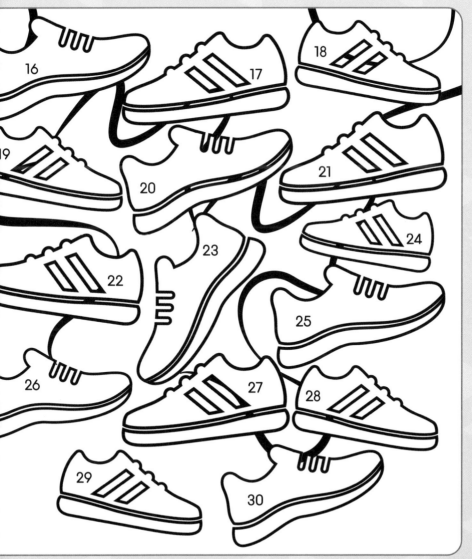

# I'VE GOT WHAT IT TAKES

# TOP TIPS

## THE IMPORTANCE OF MINDFULNESS

A healthy body is a great thing, but for our well-being to be truly balanced, we must give the mind equal priority. Mindfulness is the state of being present in the moment. As well as helping to ease worries and anxieties, this practice makes us more aware of negative self-talk, a classic challenge when getting fit. Here are a few ways to cultivate mindfulness:

- Begin your mornings with a 5- to 10-minute mindfulness meditation. Focus on your breathing, and count your breaths in a cycle from one to ten.

- When you exercise outdoors, leave your headphones at home and focus on the sounds you hear, the sights you see and the feel of the ground beneath your feet. When thoughts come, let them pass and refocus on these sensations.

- When you feel stressed or distracted, take just one minute to focus on your breath. This helps re-ground you in the present moment.

# Five-a-Day Tracker

Each apple = one of your five fruits or vegetables a day

| | | | |
|---|---|---|---|
| 1 | 🍎🍎🍎🍎🍎🍎 | 16 | 🍎🍎🍎🍎🍎🍎 |
| 2 | 🍎🍎🍎🍎🍎🍎 | 17 | 🍎🍎🍎🍎🍎🍎 |
| 3 | 🍎🍎🍎🍎🍎🍎 | 18 | 🍎🍎🍎🍎🍎🍎 |
| 4 | 🍎🍎🍎🍎🍎🍎 | 19 | 🍎🍎🍎🍎🍎🍎 |
| 5 | 🍎🍎🍎🍎🍎🍎 | 20 | 🍎🍎🍎🍎🍎🍎 |
| 6 | 🍎🍎🍎🍎🍎🍎 | 21 | 🍎🍎🍎🍎🍎🍎 |
| 7 | 🍎🍎🍎🍎🍎🍎 | 22 | 🍎🍎🍎🍎🍎🍎 |
| 8 | 🍎🍎🍎🍎🍎🍎 | 23 | 🍎🍎🍎🍎🍎🍎 |
| 9 | 🍎🍎🍎🍎🍎🍎 | 24 | 🍎🍎🍎🍎🍎🍎 |
| 10 | 🍎🍎🍎🍎🍎🍎 | 25 | 🍎🍎🍎🍎🍎🍎 |
| 11 | 🍎🍎🍎🍎🍎🍎 | 26 | 🍎🍎🍎🍎🍎🍎 |
| 12 | 🍎🍎🍎🍎🍎🍎 | 27 | 🍎🍎🍎🍎🍎🍎 |
| 13 | 🍎🍎🍎🍎🍎🍎 | 28 | 🍎🍎🍎🍎🍎🍎 |
| 14 | 🍎🍎🍎🍎🍎🍎 | 29 | 🍎🍎🍎🍎🍎🍎 |
| 15 | 🍎🍎🍎🍎🍎🍎 | 30 | 🍎🍎🍎🍎🍎🍎 |

# My Goals and Achievements

Don't worry if you don't manage to achieve your goals —
any progress is great and there's always next month!

## My goal(s) for this month

Example goal: Meditate for at least 5 minutes every day

- .............................................................

ACHIEVED
Y/N

- .............................................................

ACHIEVED
Y/N

- .............................................................

ACHIEVED
Y/N

## Steps to make the goal(s) achievable

Example steps: Pick a realistic time of day to meditate
without disruption; choose a meditation app with beginner-
friendly sessions; set a reminder for every day

- .............................................................

   .............................................................

- .............................................................

   .............................................................

- .............................................................

   .............................................................

# Healthy Weight Tracker

Keeping track of your weight doesn't need to fill you with dread as long as you remind yourself that the figures that appear on the scales are just one part of your healthy body maintenance. Weight fluctuations occur throughout the day and can be caused by many factors including hormone levels, so don't worry about small increases or decreases. The most important information you want to keep track of is your BMI, as this shows you whether you are a healthy weight for your height.

Try to weigh yourself on the same day at the same time each week.

Don't scrutinize the small numbers; maintaining a healthy lifestyle is what's most important.

|        | Week One | Week Two | Week Three | Week Four |
|--------|----------|----------|------------|-----------|
| Weight |          |          |            |           |
| BMI    |          |          |            |           |
| Chest  |          |          |            |           |
| Waist  |          |          |            |           |
| Hips   |          |          |            |           |

To work out your BMI, calculate your weight divided by your height squared (in metric). Find the BMI chart on page 152 to see the results of your BMI.

# Water Tracker

One drop = one glass (400 ml)

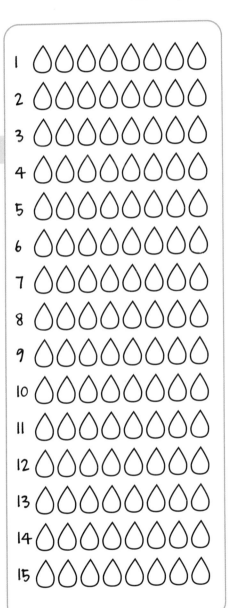

1 ◊◊◊◊◊◊◊◊
2 ◊◊◊◊◊◊◊◊
3 ◊◊◊◊◊◊◊◊
4 ◊◊◊◊◊◊◊◊
5 ◊◊◊◊◊◊◊◊
6 ◊◊◊◊◊◊◊◊
7 ◊◊◊◊◊◊◊◊
8 ◊◊◊◊◊◊◊◊
9 ◊◊◊◊◊◊◊◊
10 ◊◊◊◊◊◊◊◊
11 ◊◊◊◊◊◊◊◊
12 ◊◊◊◊◊◊◊◊
13 ◊◊◊◊◊◊◊◊
14 ◊◊◊◊◊◊◊◊
15 ◊◊◊◊◊◊◊◊

16 ◊◊◊◊◊◊◊◊
17 ◊◊◊◊◊◊◊◊
18 ◊◊◊◊◊◊◊◊
19 ◊◊◊◊◊◊◊◊
20 ◊◊◊◊◊◊◊◊
21 ◊◊◊◊◊◊◊◊
22 ◊◊◊◊◊◊◊◊
23 ◊◊◊◊◊◊◊◊
24 ◊◊◊◊◊◊◊◊
25 ◊◊◊◊◊◊◊◊
26 ◊◊◊◊◊◊◊◊
27 ◊◊◊◊◊◊◊◊
28 ◊◊◊◊◊◊◊◊
29 ◊◊◊◊◊◊◊◊
30 ◊◊◊◊◊◊◊◊

# Alcohol Tracker

One glass = one unit (recommended weekly intake: no more than 14 units)

Single shot of spirits (25 mL) = 1 unit
Alcopop (275 mL) = 1.5 units
Small glass of wine (125 mL) = 1.5 units
Pint of lower-strength lager/beer/cider
(ABV 3.6%) = 2 units

Standard glass of wine (175 mL) = 2.1 units
Pint of higher-strength lager/beer/cider
(ABV 5.2%) = 3 units
Large glass of wine (250 mL) = 3 units

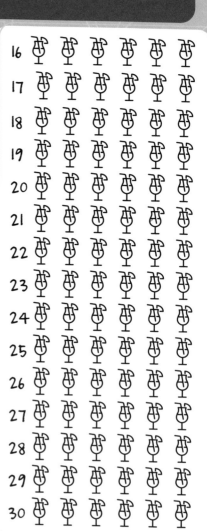

# Wellness Tracker

On each day this month, colour in one
shape according to how you feel.

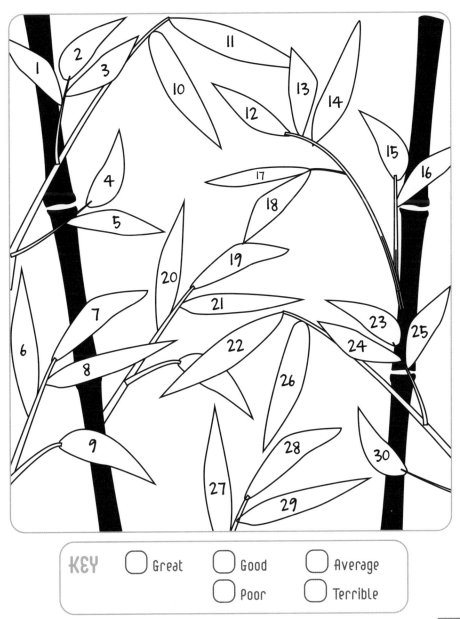

**KEY**
- ◯ Great
- ◯ Good
- ◯ Average
- ◯ Poor
- ◯ Terrible

If I do a bad
dive, that's in the
past. Move on.
It's just about being
really present in a
particular moment.

TOM DALEY

# TOP TIPS

## BELIEVING YOU BELONG

Have you ever cringed at the idea of going running in broad daylight? Perhaps you've felt self-conscious trying on workout gear or buying equipment when you're new to a sport. You can experience a deep discomfort when you feel like you don't belong somewhere but, while you can't do anything about the attitudes of others, you can do something about your own.

You might be nervous about going to a yoga studio, or maybe you want to learn kung fu but are afraid about being the only woman or minority. However, when you decide not to try something because you don't think you'll fit in, you've said "no" to yourself, and you're cutting yourself out of the picture. Instead, remember that when you head to a class or a club, you belong the moment you walk through the door. You've motivated yourself to go there, and that's all anybody else present has done. There's an instant camaraderie in that single effort.

# Exercise Tracker

Using the key, colour in and add patterns to the trainers in the space below to help you gauge how much exercise you're doing. If you feel like you're smashing it, then keep up the good work. But if you think you could do better, there's always next month!

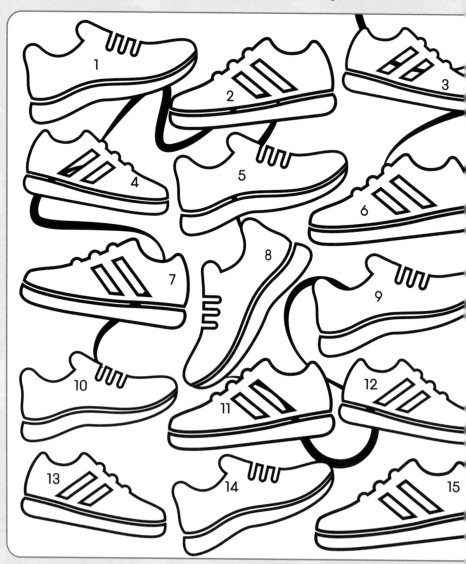

less than 30 mins

 30–60 mins

 60+ mins

 cardio

 stretching

 strengthening/ toning

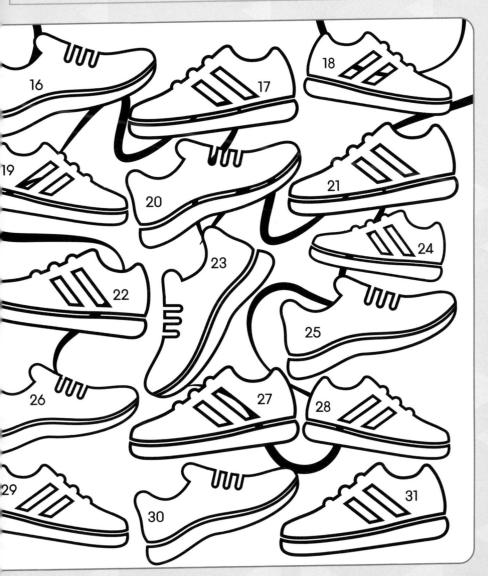

# MAKING HEALTHY CHOICES IS EASY FOR ME

# TOP TIPS

## STAYING ON COURSE

Have you ever started a new type of exercise, fallen head-over-heels in love with it and then lost all motivation? You're not alone. Here's how to stay consistent and reduce the risk of quitting.

Firstly, if you're working toward a big goal, such as a marathon, make a plan to retain your new running hobby afterward. For instance, schedule another event or commit to running 15 km (9 miles) a week. The sudden completion of a goal is a huge risk to staying on track as your driving force is gone.

Secondly, if you skip a workout, forgive yourself. Skipping a planned workout can be enough to make some people give up, but you're not a robot; life happens, and you will miss workouts occasionally. Allow it and either replace it with an easier one, or simply focus on the next workout in your schedule.

By avoiding these two traps that commonly derail fitness journeys, you can more easily maintain a regular workout programme.

# Five-a-Day Tracker

Each apple = one of your five fruits or vegetables a day

1
2
3
4
5
6
7
8
9
10
11
12
13
14
15

16
17
18
19
20
21
22
23
24
25
26
27
28
29
30
31

# My Goals and Achievements

Don't worry if you don't manage to achieve your goals —
any progress is great and there's always next month!

## My goal(s) for this month

Example goal: Stop drinking caffeine after midday

- .................................................... ACHIEVED Y/N

- .................................................... ACHIEVED Y/N

- .................................................... ACHIEVED Y/N

## Steps to make the goal(s) achievable

Example steps: Put decaf by the kettle and store
caffeinated drinks in a cupboard; eat a healthy,
balanced lunch to avoid a slump; note down every day
how well I slept to track any effects on sleep

- ....................................................
....................................................

- ....................................................
....................................................

- ....................................................
....................................................

# Healthy Weight Tracker

Keeping track of your weight doesn't need to fill you with dread as long as you remind yourself that the figures that appear on the scales are just one part of your healthy body maintenance. Weight fluctuations occur throughout the day and can be caused by many factors including hormone levels, so don't worry about small increases or decreases. The most important information you want to keep track of is your BMI, as this shows you whether you are a healthy weight for your height.

Try to weigh yourself on the same day at the same time each week.

Don't scrutinize the small numbers; maintaining a healthy lifestyle is what's most important.

|        | Week One | Week Two | Week Three | Week Four |
|--------|----------|----------|------------|-----------|
| Weight |          |          |            |           |
| BMI    |          |          |            |           |
| Chest  |          |          |            |           |
| Waist  |          |          |            |           |
| Hips   |          |          |            |           |

To work out your BMI, calculate your weight divided by your height squared (in metric). Find the BMI chart on page 152 to see the results of your BMI.

# Water Tracker

One drop = one glass (400 ml)

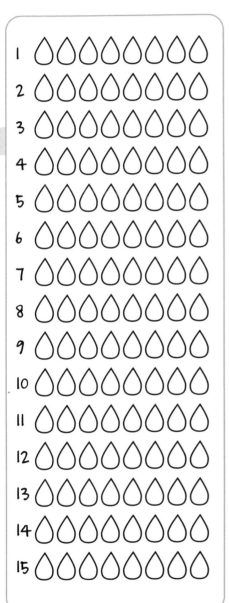

1 ○○○○○○○○
2 ○○○○○○○○
3 ○○○○○○○○
4 ○○○○○○○○
5 ○○○○○○○○
6 ○○○○○○○○
7 ○○○○○○○○
8 ○○○○○○○○
9 ○○○○○○○○
10 ○○○○○○○○
11 ○○○○○○○○
12 ○○○○○○○○
13 ○○○○○○○○
14 ○○○○○○○○
15 ○○○○○○○○

16 ○○○○○○○○
17 ○○○○○○○○
18 ○○○○○○○○
19 ○○○○○○○○
20 ○○○○○○○○
21 ○○○○○○○○
22 ○○○○○○○○
23 ○○○○○○○○
24 ○○○○○○○○
25 ○○○○○○○○
26 ○○○○○○○○
27 ○○○○○○○○
28 ○○○○○○○○
29 ○○○○○○○○
30 ○○○○○○○○
31 ○○○○○○○○

# Alcohol Tracker

One glass = one unit (recommended weekly intake: no more than 14 units)

Single shot of spirits (25 ml) = 1 unit
Alcopop (275 ml) = 1.5 units
Small glass of wine (125 ml) = 1.5 units
Pint of lower-strength lager/beer/cider
(ABV 3.6%) = 2 units

Standard glass of wine (175 ml) = 2.1 units
Pint of higher-strength lager/beer/cider
(ABV 5.2%) = 3 units
Large glass of wine (250 ml) = 3 units

# Wellness Tracker

On each day this month, colour in one
shape according to how you feel.

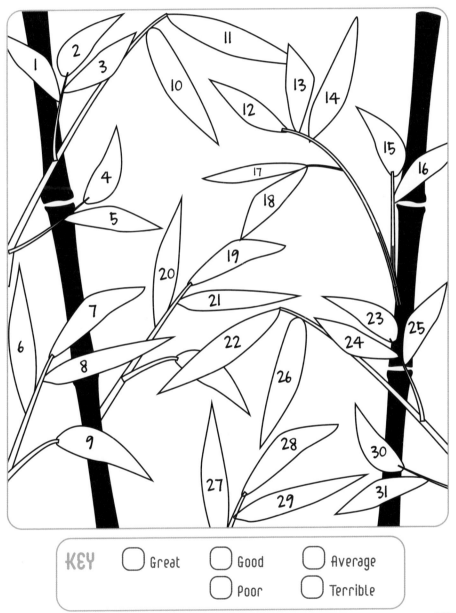

KEY   ◯ Great   ◯ Good   ◯ Average
      ◯ Poor   ◯ Terrible

Exercise to stimulate, not to annihilate. The world wasn't formed in a day, and neither were we. Set small goals and build upon them.

LEE HANEY

# TOP TIPS

## VARIETY IS THE SPICE OF LIFE

Trying new activities can do wonders for your health and well-being by challenging your mind and body in different ways. It's important to remember that your fitness journey isn't school – *you* are in control and making the choice to be active – and that just because you're an adult, it doesn't mean you should already know how to do the specific sport or class you're trying. Getting into that exuberant beginner's mindset is fantastic for staying motivated into the future.

Our bodies are designed to move in diverse ways, so why not try a variety of activities? You might just find something you love. Ever hit golf balls at the driving range? Is there a salsa class down the road? Perhaps an aerial silks studio has just opened up nearby or there are beautiful running trails near your home. From sea swimming and tennis to snowshoeing and dance, being playful in your approach to trying new activities makes it fabulous fun.

# Conclusion

This journal contains a holistic range of fitness and health trackers, so before you head into the new year, take a moment to look back through it and reflect. What have you learned from tracking your fitness over the last year? What came easily to you and what was more challenging? No matter how you found this process, it's time to celebrate yourself and all you've accomplished.

What have you discovered about yourself within these pages? Looking forward, what will you take with you into the future?

Perhaps you've spotted patterns that have allowed you to get to know yourself better or even discovered new activities you'd never dreamed of trying before. By tracking your health and fitness for this long, you will have gained a greater mindfulness when it comes to moving your body, eating and making choices for your overall well-being. This awareness can aid you in every corner of your life.

Hopefully this book has given you the space to reflect as well as provide you with insight so that you can continue your journey with a better understanding of your fitness and health.

# Body Mass Index Chart

Height — Weight

| ft/in. | cm | 90 | 100 | 110 | 120 | 130 | 140 | 150 | 160 | 170 | 180 | 190 | 200 | 210 | 220 | 230 | 240 | 250 | 260 | 270 | 280 | 290 |
|---|---|---|---|---|---|---|---|---|---|---|---|---|---|---|---|---|---|---|---|---|---|---|
| **lb** | **kg** | 41 | 45 | 50 | 54 | 59 | 64 | 68 | 72 | 77 | 82 | 86 | 91 | 95 | 100 | 104 | 109 | 113 | 118 | 122 | 127 | 132 |
| 4 ft 8 in. | 142.2 | 20 | 22 | 25 | 27 | 29 | 31 | 34 | 36 | 38 | 40 | 43 | 45 | 47 | 49 | 52 | 54 | 56 | 58 | 61 | 63 | 65 |
| 4 ft 9 in. | 144.7 | 19 | 22 | 24 | 26 | 28 | 30 | 32 | 35 | 37 | 39 | 41 | 43 | 45 | 48 | 50 | 52 | 54 | 56 | 58 | 61 | 63 |
| 4 ft 10 in. | 147.3 | 19 | 21 | 23 | 25 | 27 | 29 | 31 | 33 | 36 | 38 | 40 | 42 | 44 | 46 | 48 | 50 | 52 | 54 | 56 | 59 | 61 |
| 4 ft 11 in. | 149.8 | 18 | 20 | 22 | 24 | 26 | 28 | 30 | 32 | 34 | 36 | 38 | 40 | 42 | 44 | 46 | 48 | 50 | 53 | 55 | 57 | 59 |
| 5 ft 0 in. | 152.4 | 18 | 20 | 21 | 23 | 25 | 27 | 29 | 31 | 33 | 35 | 37 | 39 | 41 | 43 | 45 | 47 | 49 | 51 | 53 | 55 | 57 |
| 5 ft 1 in. | 154.9 | 17 | 19 | 21 | 23 | 25 | 26 | 28 | 30 | 32 | 34 | 36 | 38 | 40 | 42 | 43 | 45 | 47 | 49 | 51 | 53 | 55 |
| 5 ft 2 in. | 157.4 | 16 | 18 | 20 | 22 | 24 | 26 | 27 | 29 | 31 | 33 | 35 | 37 | 38 | 40 | 42 | 44 | 46 | 48 | 49 | 51 | 53 |
| 5 ft 3 in. | 160.0 | 16 | 18 | 19 | 21 | 23 | 25 | 27 | 28 | 30 | 32 | 34 | 35 | 37 | 39 | 41 | 43 | 44 | 46 | 48 | 50 | 51 |
| 5 ft 4 in. | 162.5 | 15 | 17 | 19 | 21 | 22 | 24 | 26 | 27 | 29 | 31 | 33 | 34 | 36 | 38 | 39 | 41 | 43 | 45 | 46 | 48 | 50 |
| 5 ft 5 in. | 165.1 | 15 | 17 | 18 | 20 | 22 | 23 | 25 | 27 | 28 | 30 | 32 | 33 | 35 | 37 | 38 | 40 | 42 | 43 | 45 | 47 | 48 |
| 5 ft 6 in. | 167.6 | 15 | 16 | 18 | 19 | 21 | 23 | 24 | 26 | 27 | 29 | 31 | 32 | 34 | 36 | 37 | 39 | 40 | 42 | 44 | 45 | 47 |
| 5 ft 7 in. | 170.1 | 14 | 16 | 17 | 19 | 20 | 22 | 23 | 25 | 27 | 28 | 30 | 31 | 33 | 34 | 36 | 38 | 39 | 41 | 42 | 44 | 45 |
| 5 ft 8 in. | 172.7 | 14 | 15 | 17 | 18 | 20 | 21 | 23 | 24 | 26 | 27 | 29 | 30 | 32 | 33 | 35 | 36 | 38 | 40 | 41 | 43 | 44 |
| 5 ft 9 in. | 175.2 | 13 | 15 | 16 | 18 | 19 | 21 | 22 | 24 | 25 | 27 | 28 | 30 | 31 | 32 | 34 | 35 | 37 | 38 | 40 | 41 | 43 |
| 5 ft 10 in. | 177.8 | 13 | 14 | 16 | 17 | 19 | 20 | 22 | 23 | 24 | 26 | 27 | 29 | 30 | 32 | 33 | 34 | 36 | 37 | 39 | 40 | 42 |
| 5 ft 11 in. | 180.3 | 13 | 14 | 15 | 17 | 18 | 20 | 21 | 22 | 24 | 25 | 27 | 28 | 29 | 31 | 32 | 33 | 35 | 36 | 38 | 39 | 40 |
| 6 ft 0 in. | 182.8 | 12 | 14 | 15 | 16 | 18 | 19 | 20 | 22 | 23 | 24 | 26 | 27 | 28 | 30 | 31 | 33 | 34 | 35 | 37 | 38 | 39 |
| 6 ft 1 in. | 185.4 | 12 | 13 | 15 | 16 | 17 | 18 | 20 | 21 | 22 | 24 | 25 | 26 | 28 | 29 | 30 | 32 | 33 | 34 | 36 | 37 | 38 |
| 6 ft 2 in. | 187.9 | 12 | 13 | 14 | 15 | 17 | 18 | 19 | 21 | 22 | 23 | 24 | 26 | 27 | 28 | 30 | 31 | 32 | 33 | 35 | 36 | 37 |
| 6 ft 3 in. | 190.5 | 11 | 13 | 14 | 15 | 16 | 18 | 19 | 20 | 21 | 23 | 24 | 25 | 26 | 27 | 29 | 30 | 31 | 32 | 34 | 35 | 36 |
| 6 ft 4 in. | 193.0 | 11 | 12 | 13 | 15 | 16 | 17 | 18 | 19 | 21 | 22 | 23 | 24 | 26 | 27 | 28 | 29 | 30 | 32 | 33 | 34 | 35 |
| 6 ft 5 in. | 195.5 | 11 | 12 | 13 | 14 | 15 | 17 | 18 | 19 | 20 | 21 | 23 | 24 | 25 | 26 | 27 | 28 | 30 | 31 | 32 | 33 | 34 |
| 6 ft 6 in. | 198.1 | 10 | 12 | 13 | 14 | 15 | 16 | 17 | 18 | 20 | 21 | 22 | 23 | 24 | 25 | 27 | 28 | 29 | 30 | 31 | 32 | 34 |
| 6 ft 7 in. | 200.6 | 10 | 11 | 12 | 14 | 15 | 16 | 17 | 18 | 19 | 20 | 21 | 23 | 24 | 25 | 26 | 27 | 28 | 29 | 30 | 32 | 33 |
| 6 ft 8 in. | 203.2 | 10 | 11 | 12 | 13 | 14 | 15 | 16 | 18 | 19 | 20 | 21 | 22 | 23 | 24 | 25 | 26 | 27 | 29 | 30 | 31 | 32 |
| 6 ft 9 in. | 205.7 | 10 | 11 | 12 | 13 | 14 | 15 | 16 | 17 | 18 | 19 | 20 | 21 | 23 | 24 | 25 | 26 | 27 | 28 | 29 | 30 | 31 |
| 6 ft 10 in. | 208.2 | 9 | 10 | 12 | 13 | 14 | 15 | 16 | 17 | 18 | 19 | 20 | 21 | 22 | 23 | 24 | 25 | 26 | 27 | 28 | 29 | 30 |
| 6 ft 11 in. | 210.8 | 9 | 10 | 11 | 12 | 13 | 14 | 15 | 16 | 17 | 18 | 19 | 20 | 21 | 22 | 23 | 24 | 26 | 27 | 28 | 29 | 30 |

**Legend:** ▪ Underweight ▪ Healthy ▪ Overweight ▪ Obese ▪ Extremely Obese

# Notes

Use this space to reflect on your fitness journey so far.

# Also Available

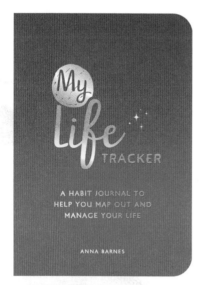

MY LIFE TRACKER
ISBN: 978-1-80007-447-7

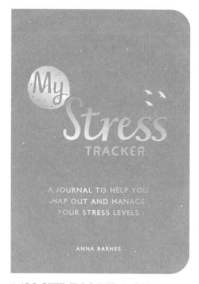

MY STRESS TRACKER
ISBN: 978-1-78783-533-7

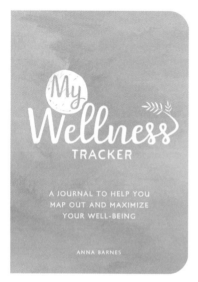

MY WELLNESS TRACKER
ISBN: 978-1-78783-638-9

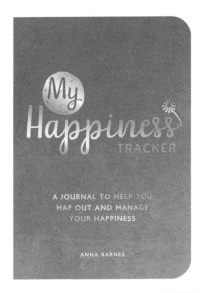

MY HAPPINESS TRACKER
ISBN: 978-1-80007-446-0

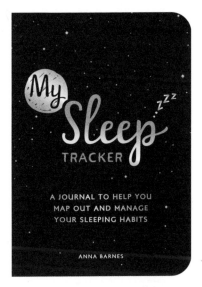

MY SLEEP TRACKER
ISBN: 978-1-78783-532-0

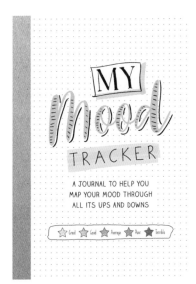

MY MOOD TRACKER
ISBN: 978-1-78783-328-9

Have you enjoyed this book?
If so, why not write a review on your
favourite website?

If you're interested in finding out more
about our books, find us on Facebook
at Summersdale Publishers and follow us
on Twitter at @Summersdale and on Instagram
at @summersdalebooks and get in touch.
We'd love to hear from you!

Thanks very much for buying this
Summersdale book.

www.summersdale.com

## Image Credits

pp.1, 4–5, 16, 28, 40, 52, 64, 76, 88, 100, 112, 124, 136, 148, 150–1, 153–7 © ExpressVectors/Shutterstock.com
pp.6–7, 18–9, 30–1, 42–3, 54–5, 66–7, 78–9, 90–1, 102–3, 114–5, 126–7, 138–9 – trainers © Janis Abolins, olahgaris/Shutterstock.com
pp.9, 17, 21, 29, 33, 41, 45, 53, 57, 65, 69, 77, 81, 89, 93, 101, 105, 113, 117, 125, 129, 137, 141, 149, © alien.art/Shutterstock.com
pp.10, 22, 34, 46, 58, 70, 82, 94, 106, 118, 130, 142 © InaKos/Shutterstock.com
pp.11, 23, 35, 47, 59, 71, 83, 95, 107, 119, 131, 143 – footprints © baldyrgan/Shutterstock.com, medals © jkcDesign/Shutterstock.com
pp.12, 24, 36, 48, 60, 72, 84, 96, 108, 120, 132, 144 © RODINA OLENA/Shutterstock.com
pp.14, 26, 38, 50, 62, 74, 86, 98, 110, 122, 134, 146 – background © Iryn/Shutterstock.com, glass © davooda/Shutterstock.com
pp.15, 27, 39, 51, 63, 75, 87, 99, 111, 123, 135, 147 © crisp0022/Shutterstock.com